Rapid Emergency and Unscheduled Care

We would like to thank our families:

Jaime and Rupert
Debbie, Rebecca and Katie
along with our friends for their patience and support

Rapid Emergency and Unscheduled Care

Oliver Phipps, MSc BSc DipHE RN
Advanced Nurse Practitioner
North Bristol NHS Trust &
Senior Lecturer in Advanced Practice
University of the West of England

Jason Lugg, BSc DipHE RN PGCert
Lead Nurse and Emergency Nurse Practitioner
Emergency Department, Bristol Royal Infirmary &
Visiting Lecturer in Emergency Care
University of the West of England

WILEY Blackwell

Library of Congress Cataloging-in-Publication Data

Names: Lugg, Jason, author. | Phipps, Oliver, author.
Title: Rapid emergency & unscheduled care / Jason Lugg, Oliver Phipps.
Other titles: Rapid emergency and unscheduled care | Emergency & unscheduled care
Description: Chichester, West Sussex, UK ; Hoboken, NJ : John Wiley & Sons Inc., 2016. | Includes index.
Identifiers: LCCN 2016001983| ISBN 9781119035855 (paper) | ISBN 9781119035862 (Adobe PDF) |
    ISBN 9781119035879 (epub)
Subjects: | MESH: Emergencies | Emergency Treatment | Handbooks
Classification: LCC RC86.7 | NLM WB 39 | DDC 616.02/5–dc23
LC record available at http://lccn.loc.gov/2016001983

A catalogue record for this book is available from the British Library.

Wiley also publishes its books in a variety of electronic formats. Some content that appears in print may
not be available in electronic books.

Cover image: Susan Chiang/Getty

Set in 7.5/9.5pt Frutiger by SPi Global, Pondicherry, India
Printed and bound in Malaysia by Vivar Printing Sdn Bhd

1   2016

Contents

Obstetrics and gynaecology

Ophthalmology

Overdose and poisoning

Respiratory

Skin

The electrocardiogram

List of contributors

Neal Aplin, BSc DipHE RN
Nurse Practitioner in Urgent Care
Carfax Medical Centre
Wiltshire, UK
and
Associate Lecturer
Oxford Brookes University
Oxford, UK

Dr Jessica Hutchinson, BMedSci (Hons) BM BS MRCEM PG Cert TLHP
Specialist Registrar in Emergency Medicine
Severn Deanery
Bristol, UK

Tom Johnson, BSc (Hons) RN
Advanced Nurse Practitioner
North Bristol NHS Trust
Bristol, UK

Preface

The growth of non-medical practitioners working in emergency and unscheduled care has been a key feature of the changing healthcare workforce in the United Kingdom. In writing this book we have attempted to cover a comprehensive range of diseases, injuries and illnesses that present to nurses, paramedics and allied health professionals working in emergency and unscheduled care environments.

The text has been designed to provide a quick reference summary of conditions, their definition, aetiology, history, examination, investigations and management. We have made the assumption that clinicians are already skilled at history taking and physical examination. We are mindful that local protocols and procedures vary and therefore regularly direct the reader to refer to local protocols throughout the text.

It has been no mean feat writing a text to cover a diverse area of clinical practice and for a wide professional audience. We hope you enjoy reading this book and that you find it useful as a reference guide in your daily practice.

Oliver Phipps
Jason Lugg

Acknowledgements

We are indebted to many people for their support and patience while we wrote this book. Many of our colleagues have read and provided us with valuable feedback on our draft text. We would particularly like to thank the following for reviewing sections of our text:

Dr Rebecca Hoskins, Consultant Nurse and Senior Lecturer in Emergency Care; Dr Rebecca Maxwell and Dr Rebecca Thorpe, Consultants in Emergency Medicine; Dr Nicola Taylor, Consultant Psychiatrist all at the Bristol Royal Infirmary; and Dr Girish Boggaram, Consultant in Emergency Medicine at Stoke Mandeville Hospital, for their invaluable guidance.

List of abbreviations

ABC	Airway, Breathing, Circulation
ABCDE	Airway, Breathing, Circulation, Disability, Exposure
ABG	Arterial blood gas
ACE	Angiotensin-converting enzyme
ACS	Acute coronary syndrome
AF	Atrial fibrillation
AKI	Acute kidney injury
AOM	Acute otitis media
ATLS	Advanced Trauma Life Support
AXR	Abdominal X-ray
β	Beta
BP	Blood pressure
BPM	Beats per minute
BTS	British Thoracic Society
CBG	Capillary blood glucose
CCU	Coronary care unit
COPD	Chronic obstructive pulmonary disease
CPAP	Continuous positive airway pressure
CRP	C-reactive protein
CRT	Capillary refill time
CSF	Cerebral spinal fluid
CT	Computerised tomography
CVS	Cardiovascular system
CXR	Chest X-ray
DIC	Disseminated intravascular coagulation
DVT	Deep vein thrombosis
ECG	Electrocardiogram
ED	Emergency department
EPAC	Early pregnancy assessment clinic
ERCP	Endoscopic retrograde cholangiopancreatography
ESR	Erythrocyte sedimentation rate
FBC	Full blood count
GCS	Glasgow Coma Score
GI	Gastrointestinal
HARM	Heat, alcohol, running and massage
HR	Heart rate
ICP	Intracranial pressure
ITU	Intensive therapy unit
IV	Intravenous
JVP	Jugular venous pressure
KCL	Potassium chloride
LIF	Left iliac fossa
LVF	Left ventricular failure
MC&S	Microscopy, culture and sensitivity
MHA	Mental Health Act
MRCP	Magnetic resonance cholangiopancreatography
MRI	Magnetic resonance imaging
NG	Nasogastric
NSAID	Non-steroidal anti-inflammatory drug

NSTEMI	Non-ST-elevation myocardial infraction
OGD	Oesophago-gastro-duodenoscopy
PE	Pulmonary embolus
PMH	Past medical history
RIF	Right iliac fossa
ROM	Range of movement
RR	Respiratory rate
RTC	Road traffic collision
SLE	Systemic lupus erythematosus
SOB	Shortness of breath
SPO$_2$	Oxygen saturations
STEMI	ST-elevation myocardial infarction
TFT	Thyroid function test
TIA	Transient ischaemic attack
TM	Tympanic membrane
U&E	Urea and electrolytes
VBG	Venous blood gas
WCC	White cell count

Cardiovascular

Rapid Emergency and Unscheduled Care, First Edition. Oliver Phipps and Jason Lugg.
© 2016 John Wiley & Sons, Ltd. Published 2016 by John Wiley & Sons, Ltd.

Abdominal aortic aneurysm
Definition
An abdominal aortic aneurysm (AAA) is defined as an enlargement of the aorta by at least 1.5 times its normal diameter. The normal diameter of the aorta is ~2 cm and increases with age. Most AAA are small and not dangerous; however when they increase in size, they are prone to rupture causing a life-threatening condition.

Epidemiology
It is estimated that in 95% of patients, AAA is a complication of atherosclerosis. Risk factors include being male, hypertension, increasing age, smoking and a family history of AAA.

History
- Asymptomatic and often detected on routine abdominal imaging or NHS screening programme.
- Patient may feel pulsatile mass in abdomen.
- Backache.
- Aching pain in the epigastrium and central abdomen to the back.
- In rupture the patient will have severe abdominal pain, often epigastric and radiating to the back.
- May be accompanied by collapse.
- Symptoms can be similar to renal colic.

Examination
The patient should be assessed using the ABCDE approach with appropriate step interventions. Specific points to increase the likely diagnosis of a ruptured AAA include:

- Signs of shock
- Abdominal tenderness and guarding
- Palpable abdominal mass – often pulsatile
- Weak or absent lower limb pulses

Investigations
- Bloods:
    - FBC
    - U&Es
    - LFTs
    - Clotting screen
    - Cross-match
- Arterial blood gas
- ECG
- CXR and AXR
- CT abdomen
- FAST ultrasound scan

Management
- Transfer direct to the emergency department (ED) with pre-alert.
- ABCDE approach.
- Oxygen (set SpO_2 target).
- IV access × 2.
- Cautious IV fluid resuscitation to maintain blood pressure (systolic ~90 mmHg or radial pulse presence), ideally with blood products.
- Analgesia.
- Early discussion with appropriate surgeons.
- Prepare for theatre.

Acute coronary syndrome
Definition
Acute coronary syndrome (ACS) is an umbrella term that encompasses:

- Unstable angina
- Non-ST segment elevation myocardial infarction (NSTEMI)
- ST segment elevation myocardial infarction (STEMI)

Aetiology
ACS is commonly caused by rupture of an atheromatous plaque in a coronary artery. This results in the accumulation of fibrin and platelets to repair the damage. This results in a thrombus formation leading to partial or complete occlusion of the coronary artery and distal myocardial cell death.

Epidemiology
Around 114 000 patients with ACSs are admitted to the hospital each year in the United Kingdom. Coronary heart disease (CHD) is the most common cause of death in the United Kingdom with around one in five men and one in seven women dying each year from CHD.

History
- Consider the history of chest pain or discomfort.
- Cardiovascular (CVS) risk factors.
- Family history of CHD.
- History of CHD, previous treatment and investigations:
- Pain or discomfort in the chest and/or the arms, back or jaw lasting longer than 15 minutes
- Chest pain with nausea and vomiting, sweating and/or breathlessness
- Abrupt deterioration in stable angina, with recurring chest pain discomfort occurring more frequently with little or no exertion and often lasting longer than 15 minutes.

Examination
- Clinical examination is often of little value in diagnosing ACS.
- It can identify alternative causes of chest pain (localised tenderness).
- Look for evidence of the aforementioned symptoms (sweating, SOB, shock).
- Full CVS, respiratory and abdominal assessment.
- Look for signs of heart failure.
- Examine chest wall for local tenderness and other possible causes of chest pain (costochondritis).

Investigations
- Vital signs – RR, HR, BP (both arms) and SpO_2
- Cardiac monitoring – to identify underlying rhythm and arrhythmias
- 12-Lead ECG:
  - To confirm a cardiac basis for presentation and may show pre-existing structural or CHD.
  - ECG changes that occur during episodes of angina (ischaemia) T-wave inversion or ST segment depression.
  - Look for ST segment elevation suggestive of an STEMI.
- Bloods:
  - FBC, U&Es, LFTs, clotting screen and glucose
  - Troponin – should be taken immediately in suspected ACS, but negative result can only be used to rule ACS at 6 and 12 hours, respectively
- CXR – useful to show complications of ischaemia (e.g. pulmonary oedema) or to explore alternative diagnoses (e.g. pneumothorax, aortic aneurysm)

Acute coronary syndrome (continued)
Management
- Refer to local protocols and care pathways.
- 999 Ambulance is required for transfer direct to cardiology in cases of STEMI for primary coronary intervention (PCI) or ED in other cases of ACS.
- IV access.
- IV morphine (dose titrated to pain with antiemetic).
- Oxygen (as required to meet target oxygen saturation of 94–98%).
- Nitrates (GTN if systolic BP > 90 mmHg).
- Aspirin (stat dose of 300 mg).

> **TOP TIP:**
> - Chest pain relieved by GTN does not exclude ACS.
> - A normal ECG does not exclude an ischaemic cause.

Anaphylaxis
Definition
Anaphylaxis is a severe, life-threatening and systemic hypersensitivity reaction to a foreign protein. Common examples include drugs, food products and insect stings. The resulting vasodilation and bronchospasm causes life-threatening symptoms.

Aetiology
True anaphylaxis does not occur on the first exposure to the allergen as the patient needs to have been exposed previously and therefore sensitised to the protein. Further repeated exposure leads to significant histamine release that increases on each subsequent exposure.

Epidemiology
The incidence of anaphylaxis is increasing in the United Kingdom and is suggested to be around 1–3 reactions per 10 000 population per annum. The overall prognosis of anaphylaxis is good. Mortality is increased within the asthmatic population, specifically those with poorly controlled asthma. Mortality rates from anaphylaxis in the United Kingdom are estimated at around 20 per annum.

History
- May be PMH of anaphylaxis or allergic response
- Sudden onset of symptoms (usually within minutes)
- Identifiable trigger (not always possible)

Examination
Patients with suspected anaphylaxis should be assessed using the ABCDE approach as follows:

Airway
- Hoarse voice
- Airway swelling
- Stridor

Breathing
- Shortness of breath
- Tachypnoea
- Tiredness/exhaustion
- Cyanosis
- Respiratory arrest

Anaphylaxis (continued)
Circulation
- Signs of shock (pale and clammy)
- Tachycardia
- Hypotension
- Cardiac arrest

Skin/Mucosal
- Often first feature
- Erythema
- Urticaria
- Angioedema

Others
- Gastrointestinal disturbance (abdominal pain, vomiting and diarrhoea)

Investigations
- Investigation should not delay resuscitation.
- Vital sign monitoring should be established (RR, SpO_2, HR and ECG monitoring).
- 12-Lead ECG.
- CXR.
- ABG.
- Bloods (including mast-cell tryptase to confirm anaphylaxis diagnosis).

Management
- Call for help.
- Lie flat and raise legs (some patients may benefit from sitting up if respiratory distress is the key feature, blood pressure is not compromised and the patient is not feeling dizzy or does not faint).
- Give intramuscular adrenaline.*
- High flow oxygen.
- IV access and fluid challenges of 500–1000 ml in adults and 20 ml/kg in children.*
- IV antihistamine.*
- IV steroids.*

*Please see the latest guidelines for specific drugs and doses.

Please refer to the latest guidelines from the Resuscitation Council (UK) available at www.resus.org.uk.

Resuscitation Council (UK)

Anaphylaxis algorithm

Anaphylactic reaction?

↓

Airway, Breathing, Circulation, Disability, Exposure

↓

Diagnosis – look for:
- Acute onset of illness
- Life-threatening airway and/or breathing and/or circulation problems[1]
- And usually skin changes

↓

- **Call for help**
- Lie patient flat
- Raise patient's legs

↓

Adrenaline[2]

↓

When skills and equipment available:
- Establish airway
- High-flow oxygen
- IV fluid challenge[3]
- Chlorphenamine[4]
- Hydrocortisone[5]

Monitor:
- Pulse oximetry
- ECG
- Blood pressure

---

[1] **Life-threatening problems:**
Airway: swelling, hoarseness, stridor
Breathing: rapid breathing, wheeze, fatigue, cyanosis, SpO_2 < 92%, confusion
Circulation: pale, clammy, low blood pressure, faintness, drowsiness/coma

[2] **Adrenaline** (give IM unless experienced with IV adrenaline)
IM doses of 1 : 1000 adrenaline (repeat after 5 minutes if no relief)
- Adult   500 μg IM (0 5 ml)
- Child >12 years: 500 μg IM (0 5 ml)
- Child 6–12 years: 300 μg IM (0 3 ml)
- Child < 6   years: 150 μg IM (0.15 ml)

Adrenaline IV to be given only by experienced specialists
Titrate: Adults 50 μg ; children 1 μg/kg

[3] **IV fluid challenge:**
Adult – 500–1000 ml
Child – crystalloid 20 ml/kg

Stop IV colloid
as this might be the cause
of anaphylaxis

	[4] Chlorphenamine (IM or slow IV)	[5] Hydrocortisone (IM or slow IV)
Adult or child >12 years	10 mg	200 mg
Child 6–12 years	5 mg	100 mg
Child 6 months to 6 years	2.5 mg	50 mg
Child < 6 months	250 μg/kg	25 mg

March 2008

5th Floor, Tavistock House North, Tavistock Square, London WC1H 9HR
Telephone (020) 7388-4678 • Fax (020) 7383-0773 • Email enquiries@resus.org.uk
www.resus.org.uk • Registered Charity No. 286360

Aortic dissection (thoracic)
Definition
Aortic dissection is the tearing within the thoracic aorta allowing for blood to create a false lumen between the inner and the outer tunica media. There are different types classified by location. Type A involves the ascending aorta and is most common, whereas type B involves the descending aorta. Aortic dissection can lead to occlusion of the aorta and its branches (carotid, coronary, subclavian, spinal, coeliac, renal), each presenting with associated symptoms.

Epidemiology
Thoracic aortic dissection more commonly occurs between the ages of 40 and 60 years of age, with morbidity twice as likely in males.

History
- Sudden onset of severe chest pain
- Pain often described as tearing in nature
- Pain often radiates to the back
- May be accompanied by collapse

Examination
The patient should be assessed using the ABCDE approach with appropriate step interventions. Specific points to strengthen the likely diagnosis of thoracic dissection include:

- A murmur heard below the left scapula
- BP discrepancy of >20 mmHg in both arms
- Widening pulse pressure
- Comprehensive CVS examination noting peripheral pulse

Investigations
- Bloods:
  - FBC
  - U&Es
  - LFTs
  - Clotting screen
  - Cross-match
- Arterial blood gas
- Chest X-ray – widened mediastinum bulge of the aortic arch but can be normal
- ECG – may be normal but may show left ventricular hypertrophy
- Thoracic CT
- Echocardiography

Management
- Transfer directly to the ED with pre-alert (ideally where cardiothoracic specialty is located – refer to local protocols).
- ABCDE approach.
- Oxygen (set SpO_2 target).
- IV access × 2.
- Cautious IV fluid resuscitation to maintain blood pressure (systolic ~90 mmHg or radial pulse presence), ideally with blood products.
- Early discussion with appropriate surgical specialty.

Atrial fibrillation
Definition
Atrial fibrillation (AF) is an arrhythmia. It results from irregular, disorganised electrical activity in the atria, leading to an inconsistent and irregular ventricular response. AF if left untreated can lead to complications that include stroke, TIA, thromboembolism, heart failure and tachycardia-induced cardiomyopathy.

Aetiology
In just over 10% of cases of AF, no cause is identified. However, common causes include heart valve deformities, rheumatic heart disease, heart failure, myocarditis, pericarditis, sepsis, electrolyte imbalance and excessive caffeine or alcohol consumption. Some drugs can also increase the risk of AF and include thyroxine or bronchodilators.

Epidemiology
AF is the most common cardiac arrhythmia in the United Kingdom with a morbidity of over 800 000 and an increasing prevalence.

History
- Palpitations
- Breathlessness
- Chest discomfort
- Syncope or dizziness
- Reduced exercise tolerance

Examination
- Often unremarkable
- Irregularly irregular pulse
- May be signs of heart failure

Investigations
- ECG – confirms diagnosis (no identifiable P waves with chaotic base line and irregular ventricular response). The ventricular rate is commonly between 160 and 180 bpm but can be less in asymptomatic patients.
- Bloods:
  - FBC (to identify anaemia and increased WCC in sepsis)
  - TFTs (hyperthyroidism is a cause of AF)
  - U&Es (to identify other metabolic causes)
  - CXR (if pulmonary cause is suspected and to assess heart failure or cause of sepsis)
  - Echocardiogram (to identify structural or valvular causes)

Management
- Refer to national or local guidelines.
- Admit if:
  - HR > 150 bpm or systolic BP < 90 mmHg
  - Any of the following are evident: LOC, dizziness, chest pain and SOB
  - Any signs of complications (CVA, TIA or heart failure) are present
  - Underlying cause requires inpatient management
- Treatment strategy focuses on either:
  - Treating and managing underlying cause.

Atrial fibrillation (continued)

- o *Rhythm control* – this can be done acutely if patients present within 48 hours of onset or electively in patients who present later than 48 hours after onset who need anti-coagulation due to the risk of thrombotic emboli with prophylaxis against further episodes of AF with medication (β-blockers, amiodarone or flecainide).
- o *Rate control* – for those patients in whom the time of onset is not known or who are not suitable for cardioversion (digoxin, β-blockers and verapamil).

Bradycardia
Definition
Bradycardia refers to a heart rate of <60 bpm; however for some individuals, this is not harmful and in fact is physiological for them. Extreme bradycardia is referred to when the heart rate is <40 bpm and is rarely physiologically tolerated.

History
- Chest pain
- Palpitations
- SOB
- Fatigue and exercise tolerance
- Dizziness, syncope or collapse
- Medication with focus on drugs that can cause bradycardia (β-blockers, calcium channel blockers, digoxin, amiodarone, verapamil)

Examination
- Does the patient look well?
- ABCDE assessment if patient is unwell.
- Full CVS, respiratory and abdominal assessment.
- Are there signs of poor cardiac output, for example, cold peripheries and cyanosis?
- Are there signs of cardiac failure?

Investigations
- ECG monitoring – to identify underlying rhythm and any arrhythmias
- Vital signs (HR, RR, BP, SpO_2, temperature) – to identify systemic effects
- 12-Lead ECG – to identify rhythm and other ECG abnormalities
- Bloods (FBC, U&Es, LFTs, glucose, calcium, cardiac enzyme, TFTs and digoxin level if indicated) to identify possible underlying causes
- CXR – as clinically indicated

Management
The focus for any patient with bradycardia is whether the rate is causing harmful adverse effects as follows:

- Systolic <90 mmHg
- Heart rate <40 bpm
- Ventricular arrhythmias
- Heart failure

Acutely unwell patient will need to be referred to an ED for ongoing care. Stable patients with no adverse effects can be managed in primary care.

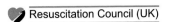

Adult bradycardia algorithm

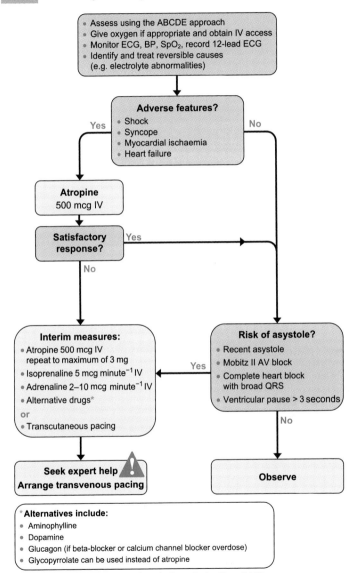

- Assess using the ABCDE approach
- Give oxygen if appropriate and obtain IV access
- Monitor ECG, BP, SpO_2, record 12-lead ECG
- Identify and treat reversible causes
  (e.g. electrolyte abnormalities)

Adverse features?
- Shock
- Syncope
- Myocardial ischaemia
- Heart failure

Yes   No

Atropine
500 mcg IV

Satisfactory response?   Yes

No

Interim measures:
- Atropine 500 mcg IV
  repeat to maximum of 3 mg
- Isoprenaline 5 mcg minute^{-1} IV
- Adrenaline 2–10 mcg minute^{-1} IV
- Alternative drugs*

or
- Transcutaneous pacing

Risk of asystole?
- Recent asystole
- Mobitz II AV block
- Complete heart block
  with broad QRS
- Ventricular pause > 3 seconds

Yes

No

Seek expert help
Arrange transvenous pacing

Observe

*Alternatives include:
- Aminophylline
- Dopamine
- Glucagon (if beta-blocker or calcium channel blocker overdose)
- Glycopyrrolate can be used instead of atropine

Reproduced with the kind permission from the Resuscitation Council (UK).

Deep vein thrombosis
Definition
Deep vein thrombosis (DVT) refers to the formation of a thrombus (blood clot) in a deep vein leading to a partial or complete obstruction of blood flow. Most commonly this occurs in the deep veins of the leg or pelvis, but the upper limbs can also be affected, as can intracranial and abdominal veins. The thrombus can dislodge and enter the pulmonary arteries, causing a pulmonary embolism.

DVT is more likely to occur in the following:

- Age over 60 years
- Male sex
- Previous venous thromboembolism
- Cancer (known or undiagnosed)
- Being overweight or obese
- Patients with heart failure
- Acquired or familial thrombophilia
- Patients with vasculitis and hypoxia from venous stasis or undergoing chemotherapy
- Varicose veins
- Smokers

The transient risk of DVT is increased in the following:

- Immobility (e.g. following illness, the use of plaster cast or other limb immobilisation devices, surgery, hospitalisation or during long-distance travel)
- Significant trauma or direct trauma to a vein, for example, intravenous catheter or IV drug use
- Hormone treatment
- Pregnancy and the postpartum period
- Dehydration

Epidemiology
It is estimated that DVT occurs in around 1 in 1000 patients.

History
- Lower limb pain, swelling or tenderness
- Can be asymptomatic
- May present with signs of PE

Examination
- Examine the entire limb for swelling and tenderness and compare to other limb.
- Measure circumference of each calf at same point.
- Inspect for dilated superficial veins.
- CVS and respiratory assessment to identify signs of PE.

Wells DVT score	Score
Lower limb trauma or immobilisation	+1
Bedridden for >3 days within the last 4 weeks	+1
Tenderness along the deep vein system	+1
Entire limb swollen	+1

Deep vein thrombosis (continued)

Wells DVT score	Score
Calf >3 cm in circumference (10 cm below the tibial tuberosity)	+1
Pitting oedema	+1
Dilated collateral superficial veins (non-varicose)	+1
Malignancy	+1
Alternative diagnosis more likely than DVT	−2
Clinical probability of DVT	High >3
	Moderate 1–2
	Low <1

Investigations
- Doppler ultrasound for medium- and high-risk patients.
- D-dimer (high sensitivity but low specificity) therefore should be used for low-probability patients to rule out DVT with negative result.
- FBC, U&Es, LFTs and clotting screen before starting anticoagulant therapy.
- ECG, CXR and ABG if PE is suspected.

Management
- Please refer to local guidance and protocols including the availability of thrombosis clinics for initial management.
- Unless contraindicated, patient should be treated with anticoagulation usually for 3 months.
- Patient should be treated with heparin until therapeutic INR is at target levels.
- High-risk patients where anticoagulation is contraindicated may need an IVC filter to prevent PE.

Heart failure
Definition
Heart failure refers to a syndrome when the heart's ability to maintain adequate circulation of blood is impaired. This results in a variety of symptoms including breathlessness and signs of fluid retention (pulmonary and/or peripheral oedema).

Epidemiology
The prevalence of heart failure increases with age. The British Heart Foundation estimates that around 1% of people aged between 45 and 64 years suffer from heart failure, increasing to 7% for people 75–84 years of age and 20% for people 85 years of age or older. Men are more likely than women to have heart failure.

History
Left-sided heart failure – Symptoms of pulmonary oedema (SOB, orthopnoea, wheeze, cough, pink frothy sputum)
Right-sided heart failure – Swollen ankles, fatigue, ↑ weight and ↓ exercise tolerance

Heart failure (continued)
Examination
- Peripheral oedema
- SOB
- Wheeze
- Cough
- Bilateral basal crackles and fine crackles throughout the lung field
- Heart murmur
- Raised JVP
- Hepatomegaly
- Ascites
- Tachycardia

Acute Left Ventricular Failure

Acutely unwell with SOB, acute respiratory distress, anxiety/agitation, cough with pink frothy sputum and signs of cardiogenic shock

---

Investigations
- Vital signs (RR, HR, BP, SpO_2 and temperature)
- Bloods – FBC, U&Es, LFTs, CRP, glucose, lipids, TFTs and troponin and ABG if acute LVF (to identify underlying causes and associated co-morbidities).
- CXR – for signs of cardiomegaly and pulmonary oedema
- ECG – to identify ischaemia, left ventricular hypertrophy and arrhythmias (may be normal)
- Echocardiogram – to assess the adequacy of ventricular contraction and ejection fractions

Management
- Acute LVF (pulmonary oedema) needs rapid intervention that includes the following:
  - Sit patient up.
  - Oxygen therapy if hypoxic.
  - Consider CPAP.
  - GTN (to reduce preload).
  - IV diuretic (if fluid overload).
- Chronic heart failure requires careful management with a clinician experienced in managing heart failure patients (GP, heart failure specialist nurse or cardiologist). Therefore patients who are not acutely unwell should be referred to an appropriate clinician.

  Management involves treating underlying causes and careful medicine management (ACE – inhibitors, β-blockers, diuretics, etc.).

Hypertension
Definition
Hypertension is defined as a systolic BP > 140 mmHg and/or a diastolic BP > 85 mmHg recorded on three separate occasions or following interpretation of ambulatory blood pressure monitoring (ABPM). Blood pressure can also be classified as malignant and typically involves a blood pressure as > 200/130 mmHg.

Epidemiology
Hypertension is very common in the western world and affects around 10–20% of adults. The associated CVS risks of hypertension have been demonstrated with various epidemiological studies, with results suggesting that for every 20/10 mmHg rise in blood pressure above 115/70 mmHg, the risk of CVS events doubles.

Hypertension (continued)
History
- Commonly asymptomatic.
- Symptoms that do occur are often due to complications and causes of hypertension.
- Malignant hypertension symptoms include visual field loss, blurred vision, headache, nausea/vomiting and acute heart failure.

Examination
- Routine diagnosis of hypertension involves recoding the lowest reading on two or three different occasions.
- In severe, resistant and malignant hypertension, it is important to assess for signs of end-organ damage and includes the following:
  CVS – LVF, ischaemia, MI and aortic dissection
    Central nervous system – stroke, seizures, encephalopathy and subarachnoid haemorrhage
    Renal – acute kidney injury, proteinuria or haematuria

Investigations
- Bloods (FBC, U&Es, calcium, glucose, coagulation profile, glucose and lipids) to assess end-organ damage and general health
- Urinalysis to assess for renal disease
- CXR for signs of cardiomegaly and if presenting with CVS symptoms
- CT of the head if cerebral symptoms exist

Management
- For hypertension with no sign of end-organ damage or symptoms, then refer to GP or practice nurse for follow-up and ongoing management.
- If acutely unwell with symptoms or evidence of end-organ damage, then refer to the medical team or ED as appropriate and in line with local protocols.

Ischaemic lower limb
Definition
Acute limb ischaemia is often due to complete arterial occlusion from a thrombus or an embolus from a proximal distal site. Without surgical revascularisation or heparinisation, extensive tissue necrosis will occur within 6 hours.

History
There may be evidence of chronic vascular compromise (chronic ischaemic pain at rest, ulcers or gangrene in one or both legs) attributable to proven arterial occlusive disease. Explore the rapidity of onset of symptoms, features of pre-existing chronic arterial disease and potential source of embolus.

Examination
- 6 P's – pale, pulseless, painful, paralysed, paraesthetic and perishingly cold limb.
- Compare pulses in the contralateral limb.
- The onset of fixed mottling of the skin implies irreversible changes.
- Check for signs of compartment syndrome.

> **TOP TIP:**
> The ischaemic limb may appear red when dependent. This can lead to a misdiagnosis of inflammatory cause, for example, gout or cellulitis.

Ischaemic lower limb (continued)
Investigations
- Doppler ultrasound may help assess residual arterial flow.
- Arteriography.
- Bloods:
  FBC – to check for anaemia as it exacerbates ischaemia
  ESR – to check for inflammatory diseases
  Glucose – to check/assess diabetes
  Lipids
  Clotting screen

Management
- Urgent admission to vascular surgeons (refer to local protocols).
  (this is a limb-threatening emergency and often requires urgent surgery or angioplasty).
- Systemic anticoagulation (usually unfractionated heparin) is often required for patients with acute arterial emboli or thrombus.
- Appropriate analgesia will be required prehospital whilst awaiting transfer to the hospital.

Myocarditis
Definition
Myocarditis refers to acute or chronic inflammation and necrosis of the myocardium.

Aetiology
It is often idiopathic, commonly due to infection (viral, bacteria, fungal) but can be immune mediated, due to drug hypersensitivity or physical element (hyperpyrexia or electric shock).

Epidemiology
Not accurately known due to many cases not identified at stage of acute illness. In Europe and the United States, Coxsackie B virus is the most common cause.

History
Presentation can be variable in myocarditis but include:

- May have prodromal flu-like illness
- Fatigue
- Chest pain
- Fever
- Tachycardia
- Palpitations
- Signs of heart failure
- Shortness of breath

Examination
- Does the patient look well?
- ABCDE assessment if patient is unwell.
- Full CVS, respiratory and abdominal assessment as minimum.
- Are there signs of cardiac failure?

Investigations
- 12-Lead ECG (may show ST segment depression and elevation or T-wave inversion)
- Bloods (FBC, U&E, ESR, CRP and cardiac enzymes)

Myocarditis (continued)

- CXR (may show hear failure or pleural effusion)
- Echocardiogram (to assess for function, wall motion and the presence of a pericardial effusion)
- Pericardial fluid drainage or myocardial biopsy

Management

- Rest.
- Focus on treating complications (arrhythmia, heart failure).
- May require critical support (CCU or ITU).
- Corticosteroids are sometimes used but evidence for use is unproven.
- Patients in prehospital setting will require admission to the hospital ideally with referral to cardiology.

Pericarditis

Definition

Pericarditis refers to the inflammation of the pericardium, which can be acute or chronic.

Aetiology

Commonly idiopathic but can be due to infection (viral, bacteria or fungal), connective tissue disease (SLE), or post-myocardial infarction or secondary to malignancy.

Epidemiology

It is more common in males and accounts for <1 in 100 hospital admissions.

History

Patients often describe initial prodromal flu-like symptoms followed by other symptoms that vary depending on the severity of the inflammation as follows:

- Chest pain (often sharp and central)
- Chest pain pleuritic in nature
- Pain relieved by sitting forward
- Shortness of breath
- Fever
- Nausea

Examination

- Full CVS, respiratory and abdominal assessment as minimum.
- May hear pericardial friction rub at the lower left sternal edge
- Occasional cardiac tamponade – look for Beck's triad (↑ JVP, ↓ BP and muffled heart sounds)

Investigations

- Bloods (FBC, U&E, ESR, CRP and cardiac enzymes) to assess for infection markers and general health
- ECG (may have widespread saddle-shaped ST elevation)
- CXR (may be normal or show pericardial effusion)
- Echocardiogram (to assess for function, wall motion and the presence of a pericardial effusion)

Management

- Treat the underlying cause if known.
- High-dose NSAIDs.
- Patients with evidence of significant tamponade require urgent pericardiocentesis.

Shock
Definition
Shock is defined as acute circulatory failure resulting in inadequate tissue perfusion resulting in generalised cellular hypoxia.

Aetiology
Causes of shock include:

- *Hypovolaemic* due to loss of circulating volume (haemorrhage, burns, dehydration)
- *Cardiogenic* due to pump failure (MI, arrhythmia or drug induced)
- *Distributive* due to the movement of fluid from normal compartments caused by vasodilation (anaphylaxis, sepsis, spinal shock)
- *Obstructive*, which refers to a reduction in blood flow (PE, tension pneumothorax, cardiac tamponade)

Shock presents in two distinct phases depending on severity as follows:

1. Compensated where the body maintains oxygenation and perfusion by deliberate changes to the physiology examples, which include increased respiratory rate, vasoconstriction and tachycardia.
2. Decompensated where the body is failing to maintain perfusion and oxygenation through compensatory mechanisms with hypotension being the key sign

History
- The underlying cause of shock may be evident (haemorrhage, burns, anaphylaxis), but shock may also be the first presenting feature requiring the underlying cause to be investigated.
- Patients often present with anxiety, confusion or drowsiness.

Examination
- ABCDE assessment and interventions
- Secondary survey guided by suspected underlying cause (CVS, respiratory and abdominal assessment as minimum)
- Identification of early signs (↑ RR, capillary refill) during examination

Investigations
- 12-Lead ECG – to identify rhythm and acute pathology
- Bloods (standard FBC, U&Es, LFTs, glucose, calcium, clotting screen) – will require other bloods guided by suspected underlying cause (cardiac enzymes, group and save, cross-match, etc.)
- Blood gas – to assess overall systemic effects and lactate measurement
- CXR – as clinically indicated

Management
Treatment should be aimed at increasing perfusion along with identifying and managing the underlying cause of shock. Specific treatments include:

- Oxygen titrated to SpO_2 levels (refer to BTS guidance).
- Fluid challenge (refer to local guidelines, consider boluses of 250 ml or 20 ml/kg crystalloid, and be cautious in cardiogenic shock).

Shock (continued)

- Treat the underlying cause of shock.
- Blood.
- Urinary catheterisation and urine output monitoring.
- Critical care review and intervention may be required.

Patients with identified or suspected shock in the prehospital environment require emergency transfer by ambulance to the hospital either to an ED.

Tachycardia
Definition
Tachycardia refers to a heart rate of >100 bpm and is broadly categorised into narrow complex and broad complex tachycardias. Causes can be varied and include medication, disease, pain, fever, hyperthyroidism, exertion, hypoxia and stimulant drugs (e.g. caffeine, cocaine, amphetamines).

History
- Chest pain
- Palpitations
- SOB
- Fatigue and exercise tolerance
- Dizziness, syncope or collapse
- Medication including recreational drug use

Examination
- Does the patient look well?
- ABCDE assessment if patient is unwell.
- Full CVS, respiratory and abdominal assessment.
- Are there signs of poor cardiac output, for example, cold peripheries and cyanosis?
- Are there signs of cardiac failure?

Investigations
- ECG monitoring – to identify underlying rhythm and any arrhythmias
- Vital signs (HR, RR, BP, SpO_2, temperature) – to identify systemic effects
- 12-Lead ECG – to identify rhythm and other ECG abnormalities
- Bloods (FBC, U&Es, LFTs, glucose, calcium, cardiac enzyme and TFTs) to identify possible underlying causes
- CXR – as clinically indicated

Management
The focus for any patient with tachycardia is whether the rate is causing harmful adverse effects as follows:

- Systolic <90 mmHg
- Heart rate <40 bpm
- Ventricular arrhythmias
- Heart failure

Acutely unwell patient will need to be referred to an ED for ongoing care.

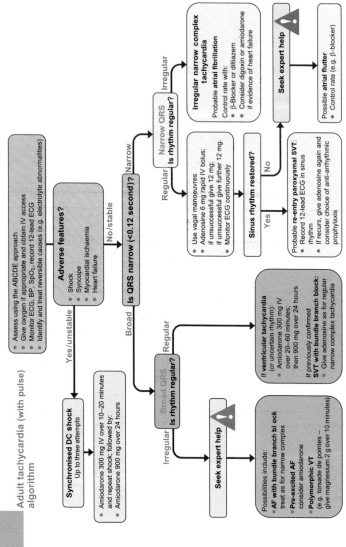

2010 Resuscitation Guidelines

Resuscitation Council (UK)

Adult tachycardia (with pulse) algorithm

- Assess using the ABCDE approach
- Give oxygen if appropriate and obtain IV access
- Monitor ECG, BP, SpO₂, record 12-lead ECG
- Identify and treat reversible causes (e.g. electrolyte abnormalities)

Adverse features?
- Shock
- Syncope
- Myocardial ischaemia
- Heart failure

Yes/unstable

Synchronised DC shock
Up to three attempts

- Amiodarone 300 mg IV over 10–20 minutes and repeat shock; followed by:
- Amiodarone 900 mg over 24 hours

No/stable

Is QRS narrow (<0.12 second)?

Broad

Broad QRS
Is rhythm regular?

Irregular

Seek expert help

Possibilities include:
- **AF with bundle branch block** treat as for narrow complex
- **Pre-excited AF** consider amiodarone
- **Polymorphic VT** (e.g. torsade de pointes – give magnesium 2 g over 10 minutes)

Regular

- If **ventricular tachycardia** (or uncertain rhythm):
  - Amiodarone 300 mg IV over 20–60 minutes; then 900 mg over 24 hours
- If previously confirmed **SVT with bundle branch block:**
  - Give adenosine as for regular narrow complex tachycardia

Narrow

Narrow QRS
Is rhythm regular?

Regular

- Use vagal manoeuvres
- Adenosine 6 mg rapid IV bolus; if unsuccessful give 12 mg; if unsuccessful give further 12 mg.
- Monitor ECG continuously

Sinus rhythm restored?

Yes

Probable re-entry paroxysmal SVT:
- Record 12-lead ECG in sinus rhythm
- If recurs, give adenosine again and consider choice of anti-arrhythmic prophylaxis

No

Seek expert help

Irregular

Irregular narrow complex tachycardia
Probable atrial fibrillation
Control rate with:
- β-Blocker or diltiazem
- Consider digoxin or amiodarone if evidence of heart failure

Seek expert help

Possible atrial flutter
- Control rate (e.g. β-blocker)

Reproduced with the kind permission from the Resuscitation Council (UK).

Ear, nose and throat (ENT)

Rapid Emergency and Unscheduled Care, First Edition. Oliver Phipps and Jason Lugg.
© 2016 John Wiley & Sons, Ltd. Published 2016 by John Wiley & Sons, Ltd.

Acute sore throat
Definition
Acute sore throat generally describes the symptom of pain at the back of the mouth, and common conditions include acute pharyngitis and tonsillitis. Sore throat due to a viral or bacterial cause is often self-limiting. Symptoms often resolve within 3 days in 40% of people and within 1 week in 85% of people, irrespective of whether or not the sore throat is due to a streptococcal infection.

Aetiology
Viral causes include rhinovirus, adenovirus, influenza, EBV and herpes simplex, and bacterial causes include streptococcus groups A, B and C. Non-infectious causes are uncommon and include physical irritation with common examples including gastro-oesophageal reflux disease, hay fever or chronic irritation from cigarette smoke or alcohol. Acute throat infections most commonly occur in children aged 5–10 years and in young adults aged 15–25 years.

History
- Isolated throat soreness and discomfort.
- Fever.
- Swollen neck/lymph nodes.
- Upper respiratory tract symptoms (rhinitis, cough, headache and malaise).
- Voice hoarseness may also be present if the larynx is involved.
- Discomfort is often exacerbated by swallowing.

Examination
- Temperature and pulse rate.
- Visual examination with a tongue depressor to view the posterior pharynx to identify redness of the pharynx and tonsils and the presence of exudate.
- Tonsillar enlargement.
- Assess for the presence of trismus.
- The neck should be examined for lymphadenopathy.
- Examination of both canals and tympanic membrane (TM) is useful in considering the presence of ear infection.
- General assessment of hydration status.

Investigations
- Uncomplicated acute sore throat does not require specific investigations.
- Throat swabs should not be carried out routinely in the prehospital setting in the management of sore throat.
- In secondary care environments, signs of systemic illness bloods (FBC, U&Es, CRP, monospot test) are often indicated to assess the extent of infection and hydration.

Management
- Simple uncomplicated sore throat requires minimal clinical intervention.
- Patient should be provided with self-management advice, which includes advising the regular use of paracetamol or ibuprofen to relieve pain and fever, the avoidance of hot drinks and adequate fluid intake to avoid dehydration.
- The use of simple mouthwashes (e.g. warm salty water) at frequent intervals until the discomfort and swelling subside.

Acute sore throat (continued)

Antibiotics are not routinely advocated. The Centor clinical prediction score can be used to assist the decision on whether to prescribe an antibiotic. Where three or four of the following criteria are present, antibiotics should be considered:

1. The presence of tonsillar exudate
2. The presence of tender anterior cervical lymphadenopathy or lymphadenitis
3. History of fever
4. The absence of cough

Admission is required if the person has stridor and breathing difficulty, is dehydrated or has conditions that are immediately life threatening, for example, acute epiglottis. Other conditions may require referral or expert advice should be sought, for example, consideration of tonsillectomy for recurrent tonsillitis.

Auricular haematoma
Definition
Auricular haematoma refers to the accumulation of blood within the external ear between the perichondrium and the cartilage, which results in reduction in blood flow to the cartilage. This can lead to necrosis of the cartilage or infection, leading to the characteristic cauliflower ear appearance.

Aetiology
The common mechanism of injury is blunt force to the ear, for example, punch or slap injury. It is seen commonly in contact sports (e.g. rugby, boxing or martial arts).

History
Direct force to the ear within the last 7 days

Examination
Examination of the ear will reveal tender, tense and fluctuant collection of blood typically in the interior aspect of the pinna.

Investigations
No investigations are required in the absence of other injuries.

Management
- Haematomas will require either aspiration or incision and drainage (refer to local protocols).
- Following aspiration, a pressure bandage should be applied to prevent further haematoma development.
- ENT follow-up should be arranged.

Referral to ED or direct to ENT specialist should be arranged if aspiration is not possible or appropriate in the prehospital care setting.

Complications
If left untreated, permanent deformity can occur, leading to the characteristic cauliflower ear appearance.

Epiglottitis
Definition
Epiglottitis is the inflammation of the epiglottis and adjacent supraglottic structures. If not treated, the condition can progress to causing life-threatening airway obstruction.

Epiglottitis (continued)
Aetiology
Most cases of epiglottis are due to infection, usually *Haemophilus influenzae* type b (Hib) bacteria, although other bacteria like streptococci, staphylococci and MRSA have also been reported. Epiglottis due to burns, chemical ingestion and foreign body should be considered depending on the history.

Epidemiology
Since the introduction of a vaccination against Hib bacteria in the 1990s, there has been a significant reduction in cases of epiglottis in children. It is now seen more in non-immunised adults.

History and examination
In adults
- Severe sore throat and painful swallowing
- Sitting upright or leaning forward
- Drooling
- Dyspnoea
- Fever
- Stridor

In children
- Tentative breathing – sits leaning forward
- Drooling or dribbling saliva
- Inspiratory stridor
- Tachycardia
- Muffled voice or cry

Management
- In the prehospital environment, if epiglottis is suspected, then immediate transfer is required to an emergency department (ED) with pre-alert.
- Management should focus on supportive measures (oxygen therapy, etc. without causing additional stress to the patient)

In the ED, the patient should be managed in the resuscitation area and immediate support requested from a senior ED doctor, anaesthetist and ENT specialist.

Epistaxis
Definition
Epistaxis or nose bleed is a common presentation in emergency and unscheduled care. Epistaxis is classified as anterior or posterior, depending on the identified source of the bleeding. The source of anterior haemorrhage is commonly the nasal septum (Little's area). Posterior haemorrhage involves the deeper structures and is more common in older patients. Epistaxis can be life threatening in severe haemorrhage or when the airway has been compromised.

History
There can be no identified cause, but some causes include:
- Trauma
- Platelet disorders
- Nose picking or excessive nose blowing
- Abnormalities of nasal blood vessels (more common in the elderly)
- Aspirin or anticoagulant drug use
- Cocaine use leading to nasal septum damage

Epistaxis (continued)
Examination
- Direct visualisation of *both* nostrils with good light and a nasal spectrum (if available) to identify bleeding point
- Examination of the pharynx to identify bleeding into the pharynx
- Vital sign assessment to assess for shock

Investigations
Bloods for FBC, clotting screen and group and save may be required if haemorrhage is severe or patient is taking anticoagulants.

Management
- Sit patient upright and forward.
- Pinch soft part of the nose for a minimum of 10–15 minutes.
- If still actively bleeding, consider the insertion of a nasal tampon.
- Refer to ENT specialist for further assessment and management, or if in prehospital clinical setting, refer to ENT specialist on call for admission or ED depending on local protocols.
- If a posterior bleed is suspected, then referral to ENT specialist will be necessary.

If bleeding has stopped for a minimum of 30 minutes with simple first aid measures and the patient has no high-risk causes, the patient can be considered for discharge if deemed safe. A further check of the pharynx is required to exclude flow posteriorly.
Aftercare advice should include:

- Resisting the temptation to blow nose due to disruption of clot
- No nose picking
- Avoidance of hot drinks
- Avoidance of strenuous activity

Foreign bodies

> If the patient is actively choking or has airway compromise, then the patient needs to be moved to a resuscitation area and managed within the latest Resuscitation Council (UK) guidelines

Definition
Foreign bodies in the ear, nose or throat are a common presentation. Adults often present to clinical settings with objects in either the ear or throat, and children often present with foreign bodies including toys, beads, foot items, etc. Throat objects can include fish or chicken bones. Insect often present with a sensation of something moving in the ear and can be very distressing for the patient.

History and examination
The patient is often able to recall the incident and inform you of the likely nature of the object. It children, it can be more challenging. Foreign bodies in the ear canal can usually be visualised directly during auroscopy.
It is often not possible to visualise a foreign body in the throat, although the patient will describe a sensation of an object. Depending on its nature or location, there may be problems swallowing food or sometimes fluids.

Investigations
Occasionally a soft tissue neck X-ray can be useful in visualising the object (if radiopaque) and for signs of soft tissue swelling. Discuss with ENT specialist first whether this would be useful.

Foreign bodies (continued)
Management
Ears
- Most foreign bodies can be removed by direct visualisation either with crocodile forceps or an ear probe.
- If the object is a live insect, drown prior to removal with saline or oil.
- If it is a penetrating FB and there are signs of injury to the eardrum or failed attempts to remove, then ENT referral will be necessary.
- Once a foreign body is removed, it is important to examine the ear for any damage or retained objects.

Throat
- If visible, then object can often be removed with forceps.
- If not directly visible or there is difficulty in removing the object, then refer to ENT specialist.

Nose
- Requires cooperation or restrain child in sitting position.
- If object can be visualised, then it can sometimes be removed with appropriate instruments.
- Other methods include positive pressure, suction and the kissing technique in children.

Glandular fever
Definition
Glandular fever or infectious mononucleosis is a viral infection caused by the Epstein–Barr virus (EBV). This virus can be passed from person to person by close contact. Glandular fever can affect people of any age but is most common in young adults and teenagers (kissing disease).

History
Patients present commonly with the following:

- Sore throat – glandular fever should be considered when tonsillitis is severe or lasts longer than expected.
- Flu-like symptoms (fever, myalgia and headaches).
- Malaise – patient with glandular fever often complain of intense tiredness.
- Abdominal pain.

Examination

- Vital sign measurement.
- Examine the throat, which often reveals inflamed tonsils with exudate. Palatal petechiae may also be seen.
- Lymphadenopathy particularly in the posterior cervical chain.
- Abdominal examination may reveal mild hepato-splenomegaly.
- Swelling around the eyes occurs in around one in five people.

Investigations
If glandular fever is suspected, a blood test for antibodies is required to confirm the diagnosis (monospot).

Management
- No specific treatment is required and the illness is self-limiting in around 14 days.
- Encourage oral fluids to avoid dehydration.

Glandular fever (continued)

- Simple analgesia for symptom relief as required.
- Avoid spread by not sharing cups and towels and by not kissing.

Mumps
Definition

Mumps or epidemic parotitis is a generalised infection caused by the paramyxovirus. The virus can infect many organs including the salivary glands, pancreas, testis, ovary, brain, liver, kidneys, joints and heart. The virus is very infectious and is spread by respiratory droplets and saliva.

Reluctance to take up the measles, mumps and rubella (MMR) vaccination has led to an increase in cases.

History

- Flu-like symptoms
- Facial swelling
- Fever
- Dry mouth (due to blockage of saliva)
- May report abdominal pain, headache, mild mastitis and testicular discomfort

Examination

- Development of parotitis (inflammation of the parotid gland) with tenderness near the angle of jaw.
- Facial swelling is often bilateral with warm and flushed skin over the parotid glands.
- Trismus in severe cases.
- Signs of dehydration in severe cases.

Investigations

Investigations are not generally required at the early stage. Mumps is a reportable disease and therefore needs to be reported to the Health Protection Agency via local arrangements. Further investigations will be arranged by the HPA.

Management

- Management focuses on symptom relief and fever and pain management.
- Further review will be required if symptoms show other organs or systems involved.
- MMR vaccination should be considered at appropriate stage of recovery.

Nose injury
History

Common causes of nose injury include falls and assaults.

Examination

- Swelling and bruising to the nose.
- Nasal deviation and deformity to one side.
- Evidence of epistaxis.
- Reduced air flow through one or both nostrils.
- Tenderness to the nasal bridge (do not forget to examine the facial bones).
- View the nasal septum and check for septal haematoma.
- Check for signs of basal skull fracture.

Nose injury (continued)
Investigations
Diagnosing nasal fracture is clinical and X-ray is not routinely indicated.

Management
- Analgesia.
- Refer deviated noses or if patient is concerned regarding cosmetic appearance to ENT specialist usually after 5 days (refer to local protocols).
- Immediately refer to ENT specialist if septal haematoma is present.

Otitis externa (acute)
Definition
Otitis externa is a condition that causes inflammation (redness and swelling) of the external ear canal and or the pinna. Otitis externa is categorised as either localised or diffuse. Localised is used to describe the presence of a boil (furuncle), whereas diffuse is caused by allergies, infections, irritants or inflammatory conditions.

History
- Ear pain, which can be severe
- Itchiness in the ear canal
- Discharge of liquid or pus from the ear

Examination
Examination with an otoscope (can be very painful) commonly reveals:

- Normal or inflamed TM
- Inflammation of the ear canal
- Visible boil (localised)
- Thick discharge (diffuse)
- Pre- or postauricular lymphadenopathy
- Mild fever <38°C

Investigations
Investigations are not routinely required at initial presentation.

Management
- Pain management with adequate analgesics.
- Thorough cleaning of the ear canal.
- Treat the inflammation and infection by topical ear drops or oral antibiotics if patient is diabetic or immunocompromised.
- Avoid promoting factors like keeping the ear canal dry, and avoid water from entering the ear, that is, swimming.

Otitis media (acute)
Definition
Acute otitis media (AOM) is an infection of the middle ear that is particularly common in young children. Although anyone can develop a middle ear infection, 75% of cases occur in children under 10. Infants between 6 and 15 months old are most commonly affected.

History
The main symptoms of AOM include:

- Earache or pain maybe worse on swallowing.
- Fever.

Otitis media (acute) (continued)

- Nausea with or without vomiting.
- Lethargy.
- Slight hearing loss.

Examination

Examination with an otoscope commonly reveals:

- Reduction in light reflection of the TM
- Bulging TM
- Typically yellow or red colour to the TM

Check mastoid for tenderness.

There may be a perforation of the TM with pus – often associated with a reduction in pain and discomfort.

Investigation

- Appropriate vital signs.
- Specific investigations are not commonly required at initial presentation.

Management

- Treat pain and fever with paracetamol or ibuprofen.
- Advise patients that AOM will usually resolve spontaneously without antibiotics.
- Consider whether antibiotics are required:
  - Most patients with AOM no antibiotics are indicated.
  - A low threshold for prescribing antibiotics or hospital admission is required for children younger than 3 months of age with AOM.
- Offer immediate antibiotics to:
  - People who are systemically unwell (but who do not require admission)
  - People at high risk of serious complications because of significant heart, lung, renal, liver or neuromuscular disease; immunosuppression; or cystic fibrosis and young children who were born prematurely
  - People whose symptoms of AOM have already lasted for 4 days or more and are not improving
- Ensure adequate normal fluid intake.
- Advise reassessment if pain is not improving in 4 days.

Peritonsillar abscess (quinsy)

Definition

Peritonsillar abscess is a complication of acute tonsillitis. Peritonsillar abscess refers to the presence of pus trapped between the tonsillar capsule and the lateral pharyngeal wall.

History

Patients will often describe the following:

- Severe throat pain often becoming, which is unilateral
- Progressive difficulty in swallowing saliva, often resulting in drooling
- Fever
- Increase in pain on swallowing
- Trismus (difficulty opening the mouth)
- Altered voice quality – commonly described as the 'hot potato voice'
- Headache and general malaise

Peritonsillar abscess (quinsy) (continued)
Examination
Examination can be difficult due to trismus; however common findings include:

- Offensive breath.
- Fever and tachycardia.
- Tender cervical lymphadenopathy.
- Unilateral bulging tonsil – commonly above and lateral.
- The affected tonsil is often erythematous with exudate and often a shift anteriorly and medially.
- The uvula is displaced away from the lesion.
- Examine for signs of dehydration.

Management
- Referral and admission to ENT clinic.
- IV access and routine bloods.
- Intravenous fluids are required to correct dehydration.
- Analgesia should be prescribed.
- Intravenous antibiotics.
- Single dose of intravenous steroids is often prescribed.
- Antibiotics alone are not usually sufficient, and ENT specialist will commonly perform either a needle aspiration or incision and drainage.

Endocrine

Rapid Emergency and Unscheduled Care, First Edition. Oliver Phipps and Jason Lugg.
© 2016 John Wiley & Sons, Ltd. Published 2016 by John Wiley & Sons, Ltd.

Diabetes mellitus: Type 1
Definition
Type 1 diabetes mellitus is characterized by an insufficiency of pancreatic insulin production, resulting in metabolic hyperglycaemia. It is previously known as insulin-dependent diabetes mellitus.

Aetiology
Type 1 diabetes mellitus is caused by an insufficiency of pancreatic insulin production, caused by damage to pancreatic islet ß-cells due to autoimmune T-cell-mediated destruction or damage to the pancreas (i.e. pancreatitis). People with type 1 diabetes are at risk of metabolic, macro-/microvascular and psychological complications.

Epidemiology
It is associated with juvenile onset, affecting 3/1000 in the United Kingdom.

History
- Acute presentations (metabolic complications)
- Polyuria/nocturia, polydipsia, lethargy and weight loss
- Incidental blood results
- Symptoms of complications

Examination
Acute presentation
Diabetic ketoacidosis (DKA): *nausea, vomiting, polyuria, polydipsia, lethargy, drowsiness, abdominal pain, confusion, Kussmaul breathing, ketotic breath, dehydration and reduced consciousness/coma*

Hypoglycaemia: *personality change, confusion, aggressive sweating, pallor, seizures, dizziness, hunger, tachycardia, palpitations, drowsiness and focal neurological symptoms.*

Investigations
Bloods
- U&Es: looking for high Na^+ due to dehydration or low Na^+ due to glucose interference with sample and for low K^+ due to cell depletion or high K^+ due to the effect of acidosis
- FBC: MCV, reticulocytes as an increased erythrocyte turnover will cause the HbA1c to be inaccurate
- HbA1c: assessment of blood glucose levels in the past month
- Fasting glucose: >7 mmol/l or random glucose >11 mmol/l (two positives required for diagnosis)

Urine
- Urinalysis for protein, glucose and ketones

Fundoscopy
- Looking for microvascular disease

Management (see local guidelines)
Hypoglycaemia
- Oral glucose gel (usually 25 g of 40%)
- 1 mg Glucagon IM
- 50 ml 20% Dextrose IV or 100 ml of 10% Dextrose IV

Diabetes mellitus: Type 1 (continued)
Chronic Management
- Insulin: many possible regimes of SC insulin:
  - ○ Mixed short- and long-acting insulin before breakfast and evening meal
  - ○ Short-acting insulin three times daily before each meal and a long-acting insulin before bedtime
- Monitoring:
  - ○ Control of symptoms
  - ○ Regular capillary blood glucose testing
  - ○ 2–3 monthly HbA1c testing
- Advice and education

Diabetes mellitus: Type 2
Definition
Type 2 diabetes mellitus is characterized by metabolic hyperglycaemia following the body's gradual insensitivity to insulin. It is previously known as non-insulin-dependent diabetes mellitus.

Epidemiology
It is usually adult onset, with UK prevalence of ~2%; increases with age and six times more common in Asians; and is associated with obesity, hyperlipidaemia and hypertension.

History
- Polyuria/nocturia, polydipsia, lethargy and weight loss.
- Incidental finding.
- Consider other cardiovascular risk factors (smoking, hypertension, obesity, lack of physical exercise, etc.).

Examination
- See 'Diabetes Mellitus: Type 1'.

Investigations
- Blood and urine: See 'Diabetes Mellitus: Type 1'.
- Oral glucose tolerance test: diagnosis is made with a blood glucose ≥11.1 mmol/l; however secondary causes need to be excluded.

Management (see local guidelines)
Hypoglycaemia
- Oral glucose gel (usually 25 g of 40%)
- 1 mg Glucagon IM
- 50 ml 20% Dextrose IV or 100 ml of 10% Dextrose IV

Hyperosmolar hyperglycaemic state (HHS) (previously known as HONK)
Usually >30 mmol/l and the absence of significant ketosis
- Refer to the hospital/emergency department (ED).
- Fluid resuscitation.
- IV insulin regime.

Diabetic ketoacidosis (DKA)
Definition
Rising blood sugars lead to a hyperosmolar state, provoking a diuretic response, ultimately leading to hypovolaemia, electrolyte derangement and metabolic acidosis.

Diabetic ketoacidosis (DKA) (continued)
Aetiology
High levels of glucagon lead to high lipolysis and increased production of free fatty acids, from which ketone bodies are derived. The ketone rise results in acidosis.

History
- Acute presentation:
  - Known type 1 diabetic
  - Unknown diabetic – first presentation

Examination
DKA: nausea, vomiting, polyuria, polydipsia, lethargy, drowsiness, abdominal pain, confusion, Kussmaul breathing, ketotic breath, dehydration and reduced consciousness/coma.

> **TOP TIP:**
> - Patients with infection in DKA may be apyrexial.
> - Consider metabolic acidosis in any hyperventilating patient.

Investigations
Bloods
- U&E: looking for high urea and creatinine from dehydration and also low K^+.
- FBC and CRP: infection markers.
- LFT: underlying liver disease.
- Lipase: could be high.
- Glucose: expect >20 mmol/l.
- Blood cultures: exclude infection.
- ABG/VBG: expect metabolic acidosis and high lactate.
- Regular capillary blood glucose (CBG) testing.
- Regular blood ketone measurements.

CXR
- Exclude infection.

ECG
- Exclude cardiac event.
- Signs of hyperkalaemia.

Urine
- Urinalysis for protein, glucose and ketones
- Glycosuria

Management (see local guidelines)
- ABCDE approach and full examination.
- Fluid resuscitation (consider adding potassium).
- Refer to the hospital/ED.
- Commence a *fixed rate* insulin infusion regime.
- Continue patient's own long-acting insulin at usual dose and time.
- Hourly CBG.
- Hourly blood ketone measurements.
- 4 hourly plasma electrolytes.

Hyperkalaemia
Definition
Hyperkalaemia is defined as a serum potassium level >5.3 mmol/l.

Epidemiology
It occurs in 1–10% of hospitalised patients, with 75% of cases associated with medication.

History
It is associated with renal failure, diuretic therapy (spironolactone/amiloride), ACE inhibitors, trauma, burns, large blood transfusions, rhabdomyolysis and Addison's disease. It can also be associated with acidosis and tissue necrosis. Remember haemolysed blood samples can cause spurious errors.

Possible symptoms: chest pain, palpitations, dizziness, light-headedness, paraesthesia, cramps and weakness
Possible signs: burns, dark urine, bruises and cardiac arrest

Examination
Nil obvious on examination

Investigations
- ECG (tall tented T waves and broad QRS)
- U&Es

Management
Mild: K^+ 5.5–6.0
Moderate: K^+ 6.1–6.9
Severe: K^+ >7.0 or >5.5 with ECG changes

Hospital treatment required:

- If K^+ <7 mmol/l with no ECG changes, repeat sample
- If K^+ >5.3 with ECG changes or >7.0, urgent treatment:
  - ECG monitoring
  - 5 mg Salbutamol nebulisers
  - 10 ml of 10% IV calcium gluconate
  - 10 units Actrapid® in 50 ml of 50% glucose over 10 minutes
  - ABG (observe for acidosis)
- Repeat U&Es.

Hypokalaemia
Definition
Hypokalaemia is defined as a serum potassium level <3.5 mmol/l.

Epidemiology
It is found in ~20% of hospitalised patients, with 3–5% causing harm.

History
Vomiting, diarrhoea, diuretic therapy (furosemide), renal disease, steroid use, Cushing's disease and Conn's disease

Possible symptoms: cramps, spasms, chest pain, palpitation, dizziness and reduced GCS
Possible signs: muscle weakness, hypotonia and arrhythmias

Hypokalaemia (continued)
Examination
Nil obvious on examination

Investigations
- ECG (small T waves, U waves, >PR interval)
- U&Es
- Mg^{2+} (if low, will make treatment resistant)

Management
If K^+ >2.5 mmol/l with no ECG changes:

- 2 Sando-K® tablets TDS for 3–5 days (max) or 20–40 mmol/l KCl in IV fluids.
- Monitor U&Es daily.

If K^+ <2.5 or <3 mmol/l with ECG changes:

- Refer to the hospital/emergency department.
- ECG monitoring.
- 40 mmol/l KCl in 1 l 0.9% saline IV over 2 hours (no faster).
- Consider replacing magnesium.
- ABG – observe for severe alkalosis.
- Repeat U&Es.

Gastroenterology

Rapid Emergency and Unscheduled Care, First Edition. Oliver Phipps and Jason Lugg.
© 2016 John Wiley & Sons, Ltd. Published 2016 by John Wiley & Sons, Ltd.

Abdominal trauma
Definition
Trauma to the abdomen can be split into two categories:

1. Blunt – compressive injury (blow to stomach) or deceleration (road traffic collisions)
2. Penetrating – stabbing or gunshot wound

Epidemiology
Abdominal injuries are the third leading cause of death in trauma. Twenty per cent of patients with significant abdominal trauma only have trivial signs.

Key points
- A life-threatening abdomen can look unremarkable.
- Fluid loss in the abdomen is often underestimated.
- Signs of injury can be late to develop or subtle.

History
- When did the injury occur?
- What was the mechanism of injury?
- Any risk of penetrative trauma?
- Light-headedness/dizziness
- Pain
- Nausea and vomiting
- Blood loss
- Bowel habit

Examination
- ABCDE approach.
- Is the patient pale – bleeding?
- Generalised pain.
- Surface marks/trauma from a seatbelt.
- Lacerations.
- Check for puncture marks.
- Abdominal bruising or distension.
- Tenderness on palpation.
- Guarding.
- Absent or diminished bowel sounds.

Investigations
Vital signs – RR, HR, BP (both arms) and SpO_2

Bloods:
- FBC, U&E, LFTs and lipase
- ABG including lactate

Radiology:
- Erect CXR
- Early CT (chest, abdomen and pelvis)
- Ultrasound – FAST scan

TOP TIP:
Cautious IV fluid resuscitation as likely uncontrolled haemorrhage. Fluid resuscitate until radial pulse is palpable. Consider blood products early.

Abdominal trauma (continued)
Management
- ABCDE approach
- Oxygen and IV access
- IV fluid resuscitation
- Analgesia
- Urgent review by a senior doctor, refer to critical care and general surgeons
- Major haemorrhage protocol if bleeding

Appendicitis
Definition
Appendicitis is an acute inflammation and infection of the appendix.

Epidemiology
It can occur at any age but more common in teens and twenty-year-olds. It is uncommon under the age of 4 and over 80. This is a very common surgical emergency with a 7% lifetime risk in the United Kingdom.

Two types:

1. Mucosal – mild form often diagnosed by pathological reporting
2. Phlegmonous – slow onset and slow progression

History
- Diffuse periumbilical pain – can be colicky
- Pain often sharp and localised to the right iliac fossa
- Alternative pain:
  - Right flank (retrocaecal appendix)
  - RUQ (long appendix)
  - Lower abdomen (pelvic appendix)
- Malaise
- Anorexia
- Nausea with or without vomiting
- Urinary frequency
- Diarrhoea (often misleading)

Examination
- Tachycardia, pyrexia and facial flushing
- Abdomen:
  - Positive Rovsing's sign (pain in the RIF, elicited by pressure over the LIF)
  - Pain worse at McBurney's point with rebound tenderness and guarding

Investigations (appendicitis is a clinical diagnosis)
- Bloods:
  - FBC – raised WCC
  - CRP – raised CRP
  - LFTs – exploring other differentials
  - U&Es – possible AKI/dehydration
  - Lipase/amylase – looking for biliary pathology/pancreatitis
  - VBG – lactate
- Urine:
  - HCG testing
  - MCS
- Imaging:
  - Ultrasound (can be difficult to visualise)
  - CT

Appendicitis (continued)
Management
- Emergency surgical referral
- IV fluids
- IV broad-spectrum antibiotics
- Appendectomy
- If appendiceal abscess (drainage will be required)

Biliary colic
Definition
Biliary colic is characterized by cystic duct obstruction or bypassing into the common bile duct. It is also described as the contraction of the gallbladder or cystic duct around the gallstones.

Epidemiology
It is often associated with obesity, an age of over 40, and a high prevalence in women.

History
- Recurrent colicky or constant RUQ/epigastric pain
- Exacerbated by eating fatty foods
- Nausea
- Vomiting
- Bloating
- Can resolve after a few hours

Examination
Abdomen
- RUQ tenderness
- Non-peritonitic
- Tenderness over the gallbladder during acute episodes

Investigations
- Bloods:
  - U&Es, FBC, CRP, LFTs and lipase – normal but exploring other differentials
- Imaging:
  - Ultrasound – likely to show gallstones

Management
- Analgesia.
- Refer to surgeons.

Cholecystitis (acute)
Definition
Acute cholecystitis is a common complication of gallstones or sludge impaction in the neck of the gallbladder.

Epidemiology
It is often associated with obesity, an age of over 40, and a high prevalence in women.

History
- Could have a history of gallstones
- Worsen with fatty foods
- Constant RUQ/epigastric pain
- Nausea

Cholecystitis (acute) (continued)
- Vomiting
- Bloating
- Feeling unwell

Examination
Pyrexia and tachycardia

Abdomen
- RUQ tenderness
- Peritonitis
- Positive Murphy's sign (pain on inspiration when two fingers placed on RUQ, not LUQ)

Investigations
- Bloods:
    - U&Es – raised urea
    - FBC – raised WCC
    - CRP – raised
    - LFTs – normal, but exploring differentials
    - Lipase – normal, but exploring differentials
    - Lactate – can be raised
- Urine:
    - HCG
- Imaging:
    - Ultrasound – gallstones

Management
- Emergency referral to surgeons
- NBM
- IV fluids
- Analgesia – opiates
- IV antibiotics – cefuroxime (see local formulary)
- Urgent cholecystectomy

Crohn's disease
Definition
Crohn's disease is a chronic inflammatory bowel disease that can affect any part of the gastrointestinal tract.

Epidemiology
It affects any age, with peak incidence in young adulthood. Annual UK incidence is 5/8/100 000.

History
- Crampy abdominal pain
- Diarrhoea (bloody or steatorrhoea)
- Malaise
- Weight loss

Examination
- Pyrexia and tachycardia
- Signs of clubbing
- Signs of anaemia

Crohn's disease (continued)

- Aphthous ulceration of the mouth
- Perianal skin tags, fistulae and abscesses

Investigations

- Bloods:
  - U&Es – raised urea or normal
  - FBC – low Hb, raised platelets and raised WCC
  - CRP – raised or normal
  - LFTs – low albumin or normal
  - Anti-*Saccharomyces cerevisiae* antibodies (ASCA)
- Stool culture
- Imaging:
  - Erect CXR – thinking perforation
  - AXR – thinking obstruction and toxic dilatation
  - CT – thinking of acute abdomen and differentials
  - MRI – looking for perianal disease
  - Small bowel follow-through – looking for fibrosis, strictures, deep ulceration or cobblestone mucosa
- Endoscopy (OGD with or without colonoscopy):
  - Assists with differentiating between Crohn's disease and ulcerative colitis with or without malignancy

Management

- Acute:
  - Refer to the medical team at hospital.
    - Fluid resuscitation.
    - IV or oral steroids.
    - IV antibiotics – refer to local guidelines.
    - Analgesia.
    - High-dose 5-ASA analogues – refer to local guidelines.
    - DVT prophylaxis.
    - Parenteral feeding may be indicated.
    - Monitoring – TPR, BP, bloods (Hb, platelets, CRP, albumin) and stool chart.
- Long-Term:
  - Gastroenterology referral.
  - IBD nurse specialist referral.
  - Steroids.
  - Regular 5-ASA analogues.
  - Consider infliximab.
  - IBD nurse specialist referral.
  - Lifestyle advice.
    - Smoking cessation and dietician referral.

Diverticulitis

Definition

Diverticulitis is an inflammation of diverticulae.

Epidemiology

It is rare in patients under 40 years. Sixty per cent of people living in industrialised countries will develop colonic diverticulae.

History

- Can be asymptomatic (80–90%)
- Abdominal cramps, often left sided

Diverticulitis (continued)
- Pain relieved with opening bowels
- Irregular bowel habit
- Flatus
- Bloating
- Rectal bleeding

Examination
Pyrexia, tachycardia and with or without hypotension

Abdomen
- LIF tenderness
- With or without peritonism
- Distended abdomen

Investigations
- Bloods:
  - FBC – raised WCC
  - CRP – raised
  - Clotting (if bleeding)
  - Group and save (if bleeding)
- Imaging:
  - Barium enema
  - CT scan – for evidence of diverticulitis
- Colonoscopy (diverticulae can be seen and other pathologies excluded)

Management
- Refer to gastroenterology speciality.
- NBM.
- IV fluid resuscitation.
- IV antibiotics.
- Analgesia.
- Refer to surgeons for surgical opinion.

Differentials
- Obstruction, perforation, abscess, adhesions and strictures

Gastroenteritis
Definition
Gastroenteritis is a bacterial or viral infection within the GI tract.

Epidemiology
Twenty per cent of the UK population will develop infectious gastroenteritis, of which one in six will present to primary care.

History
- Rapid onset.
- A certain food or meal may be identified.
- Contact with someone with D&V.
- Foreign travel.
- Recent vomiting and/or diarrhoea.
- Crampy abdominal pain.
- Flu-like symptoms.
- Thirsty.

Gastroenteritis (continued)
Examination
Pyrexia, tachycardia, with or without hypotension, dehydrated and PR tenderness

Abdomen
- General tenderness
- With or without distended abdomen

Stool
- Bloody (*Campylobacter*, *Shigella*)
- Watery (cholera, *E. coli*)
- Green (typhoid)

Investigations
If prolonged or acutely unwell:

- Bloods:
  - FBC – raised WCC
  - CRP – raised
  - U&Es – raised urea
- Stool culture:
  - Positive
  - Check for atypicals

Management
- If well:
  - Encourage oral fluids and rehydration sachets.
  - Oral antibiotics (when culture is known).
  - Antiemetic.
  - Consider notifiable diseases.
- If unwell, refer to the hospital:
  - Barrier nursing precautions
  - IV fluid resuscitation
  - IV antibiotics

Gastrointestinal bleeding (upper)
Definition
Upper gastrointestinal bleeding usually occurs proximal to the ligament of Treitz.

Epidemiology
It is more common in older adults and has an annual incidence of 50–80/100 000. Associated with acute erosive gastritis, oesophagitis, tumours and aorto-enteric fistula.

History
- Known *Helicobacter pylori*
- NSAID use
- Alcohol binges
- Alcohol dependency
- Repeated and excessive vomiting
- Acute:
  - Haematemesis of fresh or dark, partly digested blood ('coffee ground')
  - Melena (loose black tarry offensive stools)
  - Rapid bleeding – fresh blood

Gastrointestinal bleeding (upper) (continued)
- Chronic:
  - Iron deficiency anaemia
  - Positive faecal occult blood (FOB)

Examination
- Pale, cold, clammy, hypotensive and tachycardic
- Signs of chronic anaemia
- Signs associated with risk factors (spider naevi, bruising, ascites, palmar erythema, jaundice in liver disease – consider orofacial telangiectasia in Osler–Weber–Rendu syndrome)

Investigations
- Bloods:
  - FBC
  - U&Es (raised urea)
  - Clotting
  - Liver function
  - Cross-match
- Oesophagogastroduodenoscopy (OGD) to identify bleeding point

Management
- Resuscitation (direct to the emergency department (ED)):
  - ABCDE approach.
  - Large IV access.
  - IV fluid/blood products (aim for systolic of 90 mmHg in active bleeding).
  - Coagulopathy correction.
  - Consider Sengstaken tube in variceal bleeding.
  - Refer to surgeons with or without interventional radiology.
- Medical management:
  - Proton pump inhibitor (PPI).
  - Consider *H. pylori* eradication.
  - If variceal bleeding is suspected, consider vasopressin or somatostatin (see local guidelines).
- Upper endoscopy for direct management (adrenaline injection, clipping or diathermy).

Glasgow–Blatchford scoring

Blood urea (mmol/l)	<6.5	0
	≥6.5 to <8.0	2
	≥8.0 to <10.0	3
	≥10.0 to <25.00	4
	≥25	6
Haemoglobin (g/dl) men	≥13	0
	≥12 to <13.0	1
	≥10 to <12	3
	<10	6

Gastrointestinal bleeding (upper) (continued)

Blood urea (mmol/l)	<6.5	0
Haemoglobin (g/dl) women	≥12	0
	≥10 to <12	1
	<10	6
Systolic blood pressure (mmHg)	>110	0
	100–109	1
	90–99	2
	<90	3
Others	Pulse <100 (per minute)	0
	Pulse >100 (per minute)	1
	Melena absent	0
	Melena present	1
	Syncope absent	0
	Syncope present	2
	Hepatic disease absent	0
	Hepatic disease present	2
	Cardiac failure absent	0
	Cardiac failure present	2

Blatchford O, Murray WR, Blatchford M. A risk score to predict need for treatment for upper gastrointestinal haemorrhage: Lancet. 14 October 2000;356(9238):1318–21.

Rockall risk scoring system

	0	1	2	3
Age	<60 years	60–79 years	>80 years	
BP/pulse	No shock	Pulse > 100	SBP < 100	
Co-morbidity	None		CCF/IHD	Renal/liver failure
				Metastatic cancer
Diagnosis	Mallory–Weiss tear	All other causes	GI cancer	
Evidence of bleeding	None		Bleeding/clot	

Note: <3 carries a good prognosis, and >8 is associated with high risk of mortality.

Gastrointestinal bleeding (lower)
Definition
Lower gastrointestinal bleeding usually occurs distal to the ligament of Treitz.

Epidemiology
It occurs less frequently than upper GI bleeds. It is more common in older population.

History
- Bloody diarrhoea or fresh bleeding
- Suggestive past medical history (inflammatory bowel disease)

Examination
- Pale, cold, clammy, hypotensive and tachycardic (acute)
- Signs of chronic anaemia
- May have a tender abdomen

Investigations
- Bloods:
  - FBC
  - U&Es (raised urea)
  - Clotting
  - Liver function
  - Cross-match (large bleeds)
- Stool specimen:
  - Faecal occult blood (FOB)
- Sigmoidoscopy/colonoscopy
- OGD to rule out upper GI bleeding

Management
- Resuscitation (direct to the ED):
  - ABCDE approach
  - Large IV access
  - IV fluid/blood products (aim for systolic of 90 mmHg in active bleeding)
  - Coagulopathy correction
  - Nil by mouth
  - NG tube
- Surgical referral

Gastrointestinal perforation
Definition
It is a perforation of the gastrointestinal tract wall, with spillage of bowel contents.

Epidemiology
Common presentation with abdominal pain, which can be potentially life threatening

History
- Abdominal pain
- Nausea
- Vomiting

Examination
- Looks unwell
- Abdominal rigidity and guarding

Gastrointestinal perforation (continued)

- Signs of localised or generalised peritonitis
- Reduced or absent bowel sounds
- Signs of shock (pale, cold, clammy, hypotension, tachycardia)
- Pyrexia
- Dehydration

Investigations

- Bloods:
  - FBC
  - U&Es
  - Clotting
  - Amylase (can be raised in perforation)
  - ABG (increasing lactate with or without acidosis)
  - Cross-match
- Erect CXR (can show gas under diaphragm)
- AXR (can show abnormal gas shadows in tissues)
- CT scan (likely cause)

Management

- Resuscitation (direct to the ED):
  - ABCDE approach
  - Large IV access
  - IV fluid resuscitation
  - NG tube for drainage
  - Broad-spectrum IV antibiotics
  - Urinary catheter
  - Urgent referral to surgeons

Gastro-oesophageal reflux disease (GORD)

Definition

Gastro-oesophageal reflux disease occurs when gastric contents leaks from the stomach to the oesophagus that causes symptoms and possible mucosal injury

Epidemiology

Common condition, with 10–20% of adults in West experiencing heartburn, with one third having GORD

History

It is associated with hiatus hernia, pregnancy, smoking and caffeine, drug, fat and alcohol consumption.

- Epigastric discomfort
- Retrosternal
- Aggravated by lying supine
- Tooth decolouration
- Offensive taste on waking
- Relieved by antacids

Atypical

- Chest pain with radiation to the back
- Wheeze or cough at night

Gastro-oesophageal reflux disease (GORD) (continued)
Examination
- Can be unremarkable
- Epigastric tenderness

Investigations
- Endoscopy
- Barium swallow
- 24 hours of pH monitoring

Management
- Lifestyle:
  - Weight loss
  - Smoking cessation
  - Avoiding large meals at night
  - Reducing alcohol intake
- Medical:
  - Consider a proton pump inhibitor.

Irritable bowel syndrome (IBS)
Definition
A common, long-term condition of the digestive system, associated with sensitivity, causing bouts of stomach cramps, bloating, diarrhoea and/or constipation.

Epidemiology
It can affect one in five people in their lives and often develops between 20 and 30 years of age.

History
- Central and/or lower abdominal pain relieved by opening bowels
- Bloating
- Altered bowel habit
- Intermittent constipation and/or diarrhoea
- Mucus in stool
- Associated with stress

Examination
- Normal or generalised abdominal tenderness

Exclude GI pathology such as bowel cancer.

Red flags
- Acute onset
- >40 years
- Weight loss
- PR bleeding
- Anorexia

Investigations
Consider the need to investigate:

Bloods
- FBC, U&Es, LFT and thyroid function

Irritable bowel syndrome (IBS) (continued)
Urine
- MC&S

Also consider
- Sigmoidoscopy
- Colonoscopy
- Barium enema

Management
- Reassure.
- Consider medication:
    o Mebeverine
    o Loperamide
    o Aperients
- Investigate.

Pancreatitis (acute)
Definition
Acute pancreatitis is an acute inflammation of the pancreas with possible involvement of other regional tissues or remote organ systems. Mild cases are associated with minimal organ dysfunction, whereas severe cases often involve organ failure and complications.

Epidemiology
Annual UK incidence is ~10/10 000. Peak age is 60 years and it is more common in males although very common in white females due to alcohol. The principal cause is gallstones.

History
- Severe epigastric and abdominal pain:
    o Radiating to back
    o Relieved by sitting forward
    o Aggravated by movement
    o Relieved by sitting forward
- Nausea and vomiting
- Gallstones
- Excessive alcohol intake

Examination
- Epigastric tenderness
- Pyrexia
- Shock, tachycardia and hypotension
- Abdomen:
    o Epigastric tenderness.
    o Decreased bowel sounds.
    o Flank bruising (Turner's sign) or periumbilical bruising (Cullen's sign) may be seen if severe and haemorrhagic.

Investigations
- Bloods:
    o Amylase (3 x normal) and lipase (raised)
    o FBC (raised WCC)
    o U&Es
- Ultrasound (gallstones or biliary dilatation)
- AXR and erect CXR (to rule out other acute abdomen differentials)

Pancreatitis (acute) (continued)
- CT (if diagnosis is uncertain and condition is worsening)
- Modified Glasgow Criteria

Modified Glasgow Criteria (≥3 severe disease)
P (pO$_2$ < 8 kPa)
A (age > 55)
N (WCC > 15 × 10^9/l)
C (Ca^{2+} < 2 mmol/l)
R (urea > 16 mmol/l)
E (LDH > 600 units)
A (albumin < 32 g/l)
S (glucose > 10 mmol/l)

Management
- Urgent referral to surgeons
- IV access
- Fluid resuscitation
- Analgesia
- Blood sugar control
- Critical care review

Pancreatitis (chronic)
Definition
Chronic pancreatitis is an inflammation of the pancreas.

Epidemiology
Annual UK incidence is ~1/100 000. Mean age is 40–50 years in alcohol-related disease.

History
- Reoccurring epigastric and abdominal pain:
  - Radiating to the back
  - Relieved by sitting forward
  - Exacerbated by eating or drinking alcohol
- Weight loss
- Bloating
- Steatorrhoea (pale stools)

Examination
- Epigastric tenderness

Investigations
- Bloods:
  - Amylase and lipase (usually normal in chronic pancreatitis)
  - Glucose
  - Glucose tolerance test
  - FBC (raised WCC)
  - Immunoglobulins (raised in autoimmune pancreatitis)
- Ultrasound (gallstones or biliary dilatation)
- ERCP/MRCP
- AXR (to rule out other differentials)
- CT (pancreatic cysts)
- Stool (faecal elastase)

Pancreatitis (chronic) (continued)
Management
- Manage symptoms:
  - Dietary advice
  - Alcohol support
  - Smoking cessation
- Analgesia.
- Pancreatic enzyme replacement (Creon).
- Blood glucose regulation.
- Refer to gastroenterology department.

Paralytic ileus
Definition
Paralytic ileus is the occurrence of intestinal blockage due to the cessation of GI tract motility.

Epidemiology
It occurs in ~50% of patients undergoing major surgery

History
- History:
  - Previous surgery
  - Peritonitis
  - Medicines (anticholinergics, opiates)
  - Electrolyte disturbance
  - Prolonged hypotension or hypoxia
  - Immobilisation
- Nausea and vomiting
- Hiccups

Examination
- Abdominal distension, tenderness and tympany or dullness on percussion
- Reduced bowel sounds

Investigations
- Vital signs
- Bloods
- AXR (air-/fluid-filled bowel loops seen)
- Erect CXR (to rule out perforation)

Management
- Urgent surgical referral.
- IV hydration.
- NGT to empty stomach.
- Monitor electrolytes.
- Encourage mobilisation.

Peptic ulcer disease
Definition
Peptic ulcer disease refers to ulcers developing in the GI tract following exposure to gastric acid and pepsin, most commonly occurring as gastric and duodenal ulcers.

Epidemiology
It is a common condition, with 1–4/1000 people affected. It is more common in males, with duodenal ulcers often developing in the 30s age group and gastric ulcers in 50s. *Helicobacter pylori* is a common cause.

Peptic ulcer disease (continued)
History
- Epigastric discomfort
- Relieved by antacids
- Variable relationship to food:
  - Gastric ulcers are symptomatic after eating.
  - Duodenal ulcers are symptomatic several hours after food.
- Melena/haematemesis

Examination
- Can be unremarkable
- Epigastric tenderness
- Signs of complications (i.e. anaemia)

Consider signs of perforation.

Investigations
- Bloods:
  - FBC (anaemia)
  - U&Es (raised urea with GI bleeding)
  - Amylase (exclude pancreatitis)
  - LFT
- Endoscopy referral
- *Helicobacter pylori* testing:
  - C-urea breath test
  - Serology IgG antibody against *H. pylori* (confirms exposure)

Management
- Acute:
  - See GI bleeding/perforation
- Endoscopy referral:
  - Haemostasis by injection
- Refer to surgeons
- Medical management:
  - Proton pump inhibitor
- Lifestyle:
  - Weight loss
  - Smoking cessation
  - Avoiding large meals at night
  - Reducing alcohol intake

Peritonitis
Definition
Peritonitis is an inflammation of the peritoneal lining of the abdominal cavity.

It can be localised with common causes being appendicitis, cholecystitis and diverticulitis. Generalised peritonitis can be split into primary and secondary causes. Primary generalised peritonitis is associated with a bacterial infection of the peritoneal cavity without a known cause. Secondary generalised peritonitis spreads from a localised infective source.

Epidemiology
Localised and secondary generalised peritonitis is very common, with primary peritonitis being rare and usually presents in adolescent females.

Peritonitis (continued)
History
- Parietal pain:
  - Continuous, sharp and localised
  - Worse on movement and coughing

Examination
- Dehydrated and hypovolaemic
- Evidence of sepsis
- Localised:
  - Abdominal tenderness, with guarding and rebound tenderness
  - Percussion tenderness
- Generalised:
  - Unwell.
  - Severe sepsis.
  - The abdomen is rigid and tender, with guarding and rebound tenderness.
  - Bowel sounds are reduced or absent.

Investigations
- Vital signs
- Bloods:
  - FBC, U&Es, CRP, LFT, amylase, clotting and cross-match
  - Blood cultures
  - ABG (pH, lactate and respiratory function)
- AXR (obstruction)
- Erect CXR (pneumoperitoneum)
- CT abdomen

Management
- Urgent referral to surgeons
- Localised:
  - Treat identified cause (i.e. appendectomy for appendicitis and IV antibiotics for cholecystitis).
- Generalised:
  - Oxygen
  - Large IV access
  - IV fluid resuscitation
  - IV antibiotics
  - Urinary catheter
  - Critical care review
  - Surgical intervention

Small bowel obstruction
Definition
Small bowel obstruction is a mechanical obstruction of the small bowel.

Epidemiology
Small bowel obstruction occurs in 7–42% of laparotomies.

History
- History:
  - Early adhesions
  - Intra-abdominal sepsis
  - Internal, external, parastomal or wound herniation

Small bowel obstruction (continued)
- Nausea and vomiting
- Colicky abdominal pain

Examination
- Abdominal distension and tenderness and tympany on percussion
- High-pitched 'tinkling' bowel sounds or absent bowel sounds

Investigations
- Vital signs
- Bloods
- AXR (dilated bowel loops)
- Erect CXR (to rule out perforation)
- CT to define diagnosis

Management
- Urgent surgical referral.
- IV hydration.
- NGT to empty stomach.
- Monitor electrolytes.
- Strict bowel rest.

Ulcerative colitis
Definition
Ulcerative colitis is a chronic inflammatory disease that affects the large bowel.

Epidemiology
Ulcerative colitis has a 1/1500 incidence, with the peak onset age of 20–40 years. It is uncommon under the age of 10.

History
- Bloody or mucous diarrhoea
- Tenesmus and urgency
- Abdominal cramping
- Weight loss
- Pyrexia
- GI symptoms

Examination
- Dehydration
- Abdominal tenderness
- Tachycardia
- Signs of iron deficiency anaemia
- Other GI symptoms
- Blood and mucus on PR

Investigations
- Vital signs
- Bloods:
    - FBC (low Hb, raised WCC)
    - U&Es,
    - CRP (raised)
    - LFT (low albumin)

Ulcerative colitis (continued)
- AXR (to rule out toxic megacolon)
- Stool (to rule out infective colitis)
- Flexible sigmoidoscopy (to establish severity)

Management
- Acute exacerbation:
  - Refer to gastroenterology department.
  - IV hydration.
  - IV steroids.
  - IV antibiotics.
  - Consider parenteral feeding.
- Medical management.
  - Mild: oral or rectal 5-aminosalicylic acid (5-ASA) as per local formulary
  - Moderate/severe:
    - Oral steroids and oral 5-ASA
    - Immunosuppression with anti-TNF monoclonal antibody
  - Education
  - Regular colonoscopy for monitoring
- Patient monitoring
  - Regular bloods (FBC, U&Es, LFT, CRP)
  - Daily diary of bowel habits (<4 mild, 4–6 moderate, >6 severe)

Genitourinary

Rapid Emergency and Unscheduled Care, First Edition. Oliver Phipps and Jason Lugg.
© 2016 John Wiley & Sons, Ltd. Published 2016 by John Wiley & Sons, Ltd.

Acute kidney injury (AKI)
Definition
Previously known as acute renal failure, acute kidney injury is deterioration in renal function over hours or days, with the serum creatinine being more than 50% over the patient's baseline.

Epidemiology
An AKI is seen in 13–18% of all people admitted to the hospital. Older adults are particularly affected.

> Those at risk of AKI are patients with >65 years of age, chronic kidney disease (eGFR < 60 ml/min/1.73^2), renal transplant, heart failure, liver disease, diabetes, previous AKI, oliguria, neurological/cognitive impairment, hypovolaemia, malignancy, urological obstruction, or sepsis or using nephrotoxic drugs or iodinated contrast agents (in the past week).
> **Be aware of the renal effects of *all* drugs the patient is prescribed!**

History
- Severe diarrhoea
- Vomiting
- Hypotension
- Oedema
- Increasing confusion

Examination
- Overloaded:
  - Pulmonary oedema (basal creps)
  - Peripheral oedema
  - Increased JVP
- Urinary obstruction:
  - Palpable bladder
  - No/poor urine output
- Shocked:
  - Tachycardia/hypotensive and absent JVP

Investigations
Urine
- Dipstick for leucocytes, nitrite, blood, protein and glucose
- MSU
- Osmolality and Na$^+$

Bloods
- U&Es – high K$^+$, high creatinine and high urea
- FBC – exploring other differentials
- LFTs – exploring other differentials
- VBG – pH (acidotic) and lactate (raised)

ECG – tall tented T waves associated with hyperkalaemia
CXR – pulmonary oedema
Renal ultrasound
Echocardiogram

Management
- Specialist help – discuss with renal physician.
- Monitoring.
- Treat complications.

Chronic renal failure
Definition
Chronic renal failure is a deterioration in renal function characterised by a low glomerular filtration rate (GFR) and persistently high creatinine and urea. Chronic renal failure can be categorised as follows:

Mild: GFR ~ 30–50 ml/min
Moderate: GFR ~ 10–30 ml/min
Severe: GFR < 10 ml/min
End-stage: GFR < 5 ml/min

Epidemiology
The incidence of chronic renal failure in England is above 110/1 000 000 per year. There is a higher incidence in Asian immigrants.

History
- Nausea with or without vomiting
- Anorexia
- Malaise
- Diarrhoea
- Drowsiness
- Loss of consciousness and seizures

Examination
- Signs of anaemia
- Oedema
- Pigmentation
- Arteriovenous fistula
- Signs of complications:
  - Osteoporosis
  - Renal bone disease
  - Neuropathy

Investigations
- Bloods:
  - FBC – low Hb (normochromic or normocytic)
  - U&Es – raised creatinine and urea (could be acute or chronic)
  - Calcium – low
  - LFTs – Alk Phos raised
- Urine:
  - 24 hours' collection
    - Protein and creatinine clearance
- Imaging:
  - Renal ultrasound
    - Exclude obstruction and visualise structure.

Management
- Treat underlying cause:
  - Drugs: avoid nephrotoxic drugs, NSAIDS, and adjust other medicines to a 'renal' dose.
  - Hypertension – consider ACE inhibitors.
  - Anaemia – correct iron stores with regular erythropoietin.
  - Calcium – consider 1-hydroxylated vitamin D analogues.
  - Diet – high-energy diet advice.

Renal colic
Definition
A type of abdominal pain that is caused by renal stones (calculi) consisting of crystal aggregates.

Epidemiology
Kidney stones are common and usually occur in people aged 30–60 years of age. They affect men more than women. It is estimated that renal colic affects about 10–20% of men and 3–5% of women.

History
- Severe unilateral colicky pain
- Nausea with or without vomiting
- Sweating
- Haematuria
- Dysuria

Examination
- Tachycardia
- Sweating
- Nausea with or without vomiting
- Restlessness and obviously in pain
- Abdominal exam:
  - No tenderness but with superimposed infection

Investigations
- Bloods:
  - FBC – low Hb (if bleeding) and raised WBC (if infective picture)
  - U&Es – AKI or dehydrated picture
  - Calcium
- Urine:
  - Dipstick – blood seen
  - MSU
  - Pregnancy test
- Imaging:
  - CT KUB
  - KUB x-ray

> If patient is >60 years old, exclude AAA.

Management
- If stones are >5 mm, consider admission; stones <5 mm should pass spontaneously.
- Analgesia (NSAID should be the first line of treatment).
  - Consider NSAID suppositories.
  - Antiemetics if required.
- IV fluids if dehydrated.
- Refer to urologists.

Testicular torsion
Definition
Testicular torsion is defined as the twisting or torsion of the spermatic cord that results in venous outflow obstruction from the testis and then progressing to arterial occlusion leading to testicular infarction.

Testicular torsion (continued)
Epidemiology
It has an approximately 1/4000 annual incidence and is the most common cause of acute scrotal pain in 10–18-year-olds.

History
- Sudden onset
- Severe pain
- Similar pain previously
- Can awake from sleep
- Abdominal pain
- Nausea with or without vomiting

Examination
- Scrotal swelling on the affected side and maybe erythematous.
- Affected testis lying higher than the contralateral side.
- Thickened cord may be palpable.
- Cremasteric reflex may be absent.

> An acutely tender and swollen testis in a young boy or adolescent should be treated as torsion and urgent exploration is required.

Investigations
- Doppler or Duplex imaging of the testis

Management
- Urgent referral to surgeons, ideally within 6 hours of onset

Urinary tract infection (UTI)
Definition
It is an infection of the urinary tract that can affect the bladder, kidneys or prostate.

Epidemiology
It is more common in females, with 50% of all women in the United Kingdom having UTI at least once in their lives. 1 in 2000 healthy men will develop UTI each year. UTIs can be found in 5% of pregnant females.

History
- Can be asymptomatic
- Frequency
- Burning sensation on micturition
- Haematuria
- Suprapubic pain
- Loin pain
- Flu-like symptoms
- Pyrexia
- Retention or poor flow (prostatitis)
- Confusion and incontinence in the elderly

Examination
- Nil on examination.
- Suprapubic pain may be present.
- Tachycardia.

Urinary tract infection (UTI) (continued)
- Hypotensive.
- Renal angle tenderness.
- Pyrexia.

Investigations
If prolonged illness or systemically unwell:

- Bloods:
    - FBC – raised WBC
    - U&Es – possible AKI or dehydrated picture
    - CRP – raised
    - VBG (lactate) – could be raised
    - Blood cultures
- Urine:
    - Dipstick – infective picture
    - MSU
    - Pregnancy test

Management
- Consider oral antibiotics and oral hydration.
- Admit if unwell and/or dehydrated (think sepsis six).
    - IV fluids
    - IV antibiotics

Infections, sepsis and infectious diseases

Rapid Emergency and Unscheduled Care, First Edition. Oliver Phipps and Jason Lugg.
© 2016 John Wiley & Sons, Ltd. Published 2016 by John Wiley & Sons, Ltd.

Malaria

Definition

Malaria is a protozoan infection transmitted by anopheline mosquitoes and is the most important parasitic disease in humans. It is one of the most common causes of fever and illnesses in the tropics.

Epidemiology

Three billion people in endemic areas are at risk of malaria, and ~500 million clinical cases occur annually, with between one and three million deaths annually (a large number are African infants).

	Incubation	Symptoms
Plasmodium vivax	10–17 days	Within 48 hours
Plasmodium ovale	10–17 days	
Plasmodium malariae	18–40 days	Within 72 hours
Plasmodium falciparum	7–10 days	36–48 hours

> **TOP TIP:**
> Always check for malaria in any sick patient from an endemic area. Suspect any foreign traveller who presents with unexplained illness within 2 months of travel to endemic area.

History

- Foreign travel to endemic area
- Fever
- Flu-like symptoms:
  - Headache, malaise and myalgia
  - Aching
  - Diarrhoea

> In children, malaria may be misleading with fever, cough, D&V, anaemia and hypoglycaemia.

Examination

- Dehydrated with or without shock
- Visible shaking (paroxysm rigour)
- Sweating
- Fever (>40°C) – peaking every third day
- Anaemia
- Jaundice
- Hepatosplenomegaly

Malaria (continued)

> **Severe**
> Cerebral malaria:
> - Coma and seizures
> - Oculogyric crisis
> - Focal neurology
> Cardiac failure
> Pulmonary oedema

Investigations
Bloods
- Malaria parasites
- U&Es (dehydration and AKI may develop)
- FBC (low Hb, neutropenia, thrombocytopenia)
- Blood glucose (severe hypoglycaemia)

Urine
- Haemolysis ('blackwater fever')

Management
- Admit to the hospital.
- If acutely unwell, apply the ABCDE approach.
- Discuss with infectious disease specialist.
- Consider treatment:
  - Artesunate
  - Quinine-based drugs
- Paracetamol for fever
- IV fluid rehydration
- Blood glucose monitoring
- Daily parasite count
- Daily bloods (U&E, LFT, FBC)

Sepsis
Definition
Sepsis is a time-critical condition caused by the body's immune response to infection and can lead to septic shock, organ damage, multi-organ failure and death.

Sepsis causes a number of abnormal physiological processes, which include:

- Abnormal coagulation
- Neutrophil hyperactivity
- Poor glycaemic control
- Reduction in steroid hormones

Epidemiology
It is estimated that sepsis is responsible for around 100 000 emergency admissions and around 40 000 deaths annually in the United Kingdom.

History
- May have been unwell in days preceding consultation
- May have been seen by clinician recently and not responding to treatment and may be deteriorating

Sepsis (continued)
- May have deteriorated rapidly
- May have non-specific symptoms, for example, nausea and vomiting, abdominal pain and lethargy

Examination
- ABCDE assessment and interventions
- Secondary survey guided by suspected underlying cause of sepsis (CVS, respiratory and abdominal assessment as minimum)

Step 1	Assess for signs of sepsis: does the patient have systemic inflammatory response syndrome (SIRS)? SIRS criteria:	
	Temperature <36 or >38 Heart rate >90 Respiratory rate >20 Acutely altered mental state WCC <4 or >12 Glucose >7.7 in nondiabetic	Two or more of the aforementioned criteria indicate the patient is positive for SIRS
Step 2	Does the patient have signs of new sepsis:	
	Cough/sputum/chest pain Abdominal pain/distension/diarrhoea Headache with neck stiffness Dysuria Cellulitis/wound infection/septic arthritis	If yes to any evidence of new infection, then the patient *has* sepsis • Commence sepsis six as per 'Management' section

Investigations
- Vital signs (HR, RR, BP, SpO$_2$, temp) – to aid the identification of causes and systemic effects
- Bloods (standard FBC, U&Es, LFTs, glucose, calcium, clotting screen)
- Blood gas – to assess overall systemic effects and lactate measurement
- CXR and other imaging – as clinically indicated
- 12-Lead ECG – to identify rhythm and acute pathology

Management
Commence sepsis six – target within 1 hour:

1. High-flow oxygen therapy (caution if COPD).
2. Blood cultures (ideally prior to antibiotics).
3. IV antibiotics (refer to local guidelines).
4. Fluid challenge (crystalloid 500 ml if normotensive, if systolic BP<90, 20 ml/kg).
5. Measure lactate.
6. Measure urine output – consider catheterisation.

Patients with identified or suspected sepsis in the prehospital environment require emergency transfer by ambulance to the hospital to an emergency department

Septic arthritis
Definition
Septic arthritis is inflammation of a joint caused by a bacterial infection.

Epidemiology
Septic arthritis can be seen at any age, including in babies and infants, although it is less common in older children, teenagers and young adults.

Septic arthritis (continued)

Risk factors
- Known joint disease
- Prosthetic joint
- Immunosuppression
- Known diabetes

History
- Rapid onset of single painful joint
- Fever

Examination
- Held slightly flexed
- Swollen
- Warm to touch
- Tender on palpation
- Red
- Pain on active and passive movement
- Reduced ROM

Investigations
Bloods
- WCC raised
- CRP raised
- Positive blood culture

Joint aspiration
- Positive white cell count
- Positive culture

X-ray
- Baseline

Likely organisms: staph, strep, *Haemophilus* and TB

Management
- Analgesia
- Urgent orthopaedic referral
- IV antibiotics for ≥6 weeks (after diagnostic aspiration)
- May require daily aspiration

TOP TIP:
- A septic arthritis cannot be excluded by being able to move a joint passively.
- An abnormal joint is prone to infection.

Typhoid
Definition
Typhoid fever, also known simply as typhoid, is a symptomatic bacterial infection that can spread throughout the body.

Typhoid (continued)
Epidemiology
It is an enteric fever, following infection with *Salmonella*, which is endemic. Transmission is via ingestion of contaminated food or water.

History
- Headache
- Fever
- Dry cough
- Abdominal pain
- Constipation (may have diarrhoea)
- Confusion and hallucinations

Examination
- May be normal
- Relative bradycardia (15–20 bpm below expected pulse)
- 'Rose spots' on the lower chest/upper abdomen, which blanch on pressure
- Dehydration
- Respiratory symptoms (pneumonia/LRTI)
- Signs of GI bleeding

> Note: incubation is 10–20 days; if untreated, it can last ~4 weeks.

Investigations
- Bloods:
    - FBC (leucopenia)
    - Malaria blood films
    - U&E
    - CRP
    - Blood cultures
- CXR (for pneumonia/TB signs)

Management
- Urgent referral to an infectious diseases unit.
- Isolation and barrier nursing.
- IV antibiotics (usually a triple therapy combination).
- IV steroids.
- IV hydration.
- Inform HPA (tel: 020 8327 6017).

Mental health emergencies

Mental health overview

Patients attending emergency and unscheduled care settings with acute or chronic mental health conditions are common presentations. Patients often present with acute mental health crisis with or without the presence of other agencies (e.g. support workers, police).

Emergency and unscheduled care environment vary considerably in the resources available to care for patients with mental health emergencies. This fast-paced and often noisy clinical area can inevitably lead to increased anxiety for patients and their carers. Many Emergency Departments have dedicated mental health liaison services that contribute significantly to the care provided to patients suffering with mental health illness. The roles of emergency and unscheduled care environments include:

- Stabilisation of the aroused or frightened patient
- Management of behavioural disturbance in the ED
- Exclusion of medical causes for the psychiatric presentation
- Assessment of the presence of co-morbid medical illness
- Arrangement of referral to mental health services

The importance of a robust initial assessment cannot be overstated. Often performed at the triage stage, it is essential to ascertain the extent of the presentation and the level of risk to the patient themselves and others. Many environments use mental health assessment matrix that assists with identifying risk and urgency for non-mental health trained clinicians.

Specific points for assessment include the following:

- Ensure another member of the staff is aware or present if there are concerns regarding safety.
- Staff should be calm and aim to put the patient at ease with open body language and good eye contact maintained.
- Do not be afraid to ask probing questions and to enquire about expectations.
- Consider organic causes for behaviour (recreational drugs, infection, metabolic disturbance, etc.).
- In cases of self-harm ask what the patient's intention was at the time and their mood now.

The assessment should identify:

- Presenting problem
- Social circumstances
- Current or previous treatment
- Current or past engagement with mental health services
- Current medication
- Alcohol or drug use

The mental status examination provides a useful aid memoire when assessing mental health patients and equally provides a good structure when documenting your assessment.

The mental status examination is as follows:

General appearance:
- Appearance
  - Co-operative
  - Friendly, eye contact, confused, alert
  - Clothing
  - Hygiene and grooming
  - Facial expression

Psychomotor:
- Gait
  - Posture
  - Rate of movements
  - Coordination
  - Abnormal movements

(Continued)

Mental health overview (continued)

Mood and affect:
- Depressed, euphoric or suspicious
  - Range and intensity
  - Appropriateness
  - Mood or feelings
  - Anxiety

Speech:
- Rate
  - Flow
  - Volume
  - Clarity
  - Quantity
  - Liveliness

Cognition:
- Attention and concentration
  - Memory
  - Insight
  - Orientation
  - Judgement

Thought patterns:
- Flight of ideas
  - Clarity
  - Relevance
  - Flow
  - Content
  - Continuity of thought
  - Delusional
  - Suicidal

Insight:
- Capacity to understand symptoms
  - Knowledge of illness and medication
  - Compliance with treatment

Characteristics of different psychiatric illnesses
Borderline personality disorder
- Rigid fixed perception of the world
- Commonly occurs in individuals with traumatic childhoods
- Extreme fear of abandonment
- Chaotic relationships, emotional dysregulation and intense reactions to situations
- Dramatic, manipulative and attention-seeking behaviours
- Self-harm behaviours (e.g. cutting) used to manage intense feelings
- Can be chronically suicidal

Bipolar disorder
- Also known as manic depressive illness.
- Characterised by extreme mood swings and behaviours.
- Affect during mania can be either euphoric or irritable.
- Mania characterised by delusional thinking, rapid and pressured speech and often impulsive risky behaviours.

Psychosis/schizophrenia
- Characterised by delusions, disorganisation in thinking and hallucinations.
- Psychosis (unrelated to schizophrenia) can be short term, drug induced, caused by medical issues or related to other mental illnesses, for example, bipolar disorder or major depression.
- Schizophrenia onset is typically during adolescence or young adulthood.
- Schizophrenia is caused by a disruption in brain chemistry.
- Patients with schizophrenia can be very frightened and anxious.
- New-onset psychosis needs medical workup.

Characteristics of different psychiatric illnesses (continued)
Depression
- Can be acute major depressive episode or chronic (dysthymia).
- Major depressive disorder can be a progressive illness, which will worsen if left untreated.
- Multiple issues, for example, medical problems, relationship difficulties, financial troubles and ageing, can be stressors.
- Physical symptoms can include fatigue, nausea and headaches.
- Some patients will present wanting connection to services, hospitalisation or treatment for medical issue related to depression.

Anxiety/anxiety disorders
- Anxiety is a more difficult emotion to handle than anger or depression.
- Symptoms can be overwhelming to patients.
- Patients may have difficulty making decisions and be unco-operative or irrational.
- During panic attacks, patients are unable to process what is being said to them.
- Anxiety is a strong component of many other psychiatric disorders.
- Physical symptoms include nausea, chest pain, shortness of breath, dizziness and headaches.

Acute confusion (delirium)
Definition
Delirium is a clinical syndrome that is difficult to define. It involves abnormalities in the patients thought, level of awareness and perception. It commonly is of acute onset and can be intermittent in nature. It is a common presentation, particularly in the elderly, although it can occur at any age. Delirium accounts for around 15–20% of all general admissions to hospital. The incidence of delirium is also higher in those patients with a pre-existing cognitive impairment.

History
- Relatives and carers will often describe the patient as being acutely confused.
- Confusion can be associated with evident physical illness.
- Confusion can be acute or sub-acute and even intermittent.

There are many diverse causes, which include:

- Acute infections (UTI, sepsis, pneumonia)
- Prescribed drugs (benzodiazepines, analgesics, anticonvulsants, Parkinson's medications)
- Post-operative patients
- Toxic substances (substance misuse or withdrawal; alcohol – acute intoxication or withdrawal)
- Cerebrovascular haemorrhage or infarction
- Cardiac failure or ischaemia
- Hypoxia
- Electrolyte abnormalities (hyponatraemia, hypercalcaemia)
- Hypoglycaemia or hyperglycaemia
- Hepatic impairment
- Renal impairment
- Trauma (head injury)
- Urinary retention
- Constipation and faecal impaction

Acute confusion (delirium) (continued)
Examination
The examination of the patient should focus on identifying the cause of the acute confusion. The minimum examination should include the following:

- Check ABC.
- Check conscious level (AVPU or GCS).
- Record vital signs (respiratory rate, pulse oximetry, pulse, blood pressure, temperature).
- Check capillary blood glucose.
- Perform full cardiovascular, respiratory, abdominal and neurological examination.
- Perform genitourinary examination (if appropriate).

Further tests will be required as appropriate and include:

- Looking for sources of infection, including the ears and throat, rashes and lymphadenopathy
- Checking for constipation
- Bloods (FBC, U&Es, glucose, calcium, magnesium, LFTs, TFTs, cardiac enzymes)
- Urine dipstick testing and microscopy
- Blood cultures if indicated
- ECG
- Chest X-ray and possibly abdominal X-ray if indicated
- Further imaging to be considered, for example, CT head

Management
- Management of acute confusion focuses on identifying the underlying cause and treating appropriately.
- Hospital admission is often necessary to access the tests required.
- Patient safety needs to be considered paramount in deciding to treat within the community in conjunction with confidence in diagnosing the underlying cause.
- Managing confused patients should always focus on controlling the environment, familiar faces and one to one care where possible.
- The use of drug therapy to treat delirium can lead to further adverse effects and the worsening of delirium; therefore careful consideration is required. Drugs like haloperidol are the preferred first choice. If alcohol withdrawal is considered the cause of delirium, a benzodiazepine such as diazepam or chlordiazepoxide is the preferred choice.

Acute psychosis
Definition
This is a common psychiatric presentation in emergency and unscheduled care settings. It can represent a manifestation of an underlying psychiatric condition but may also be caused by recreational drug use or due to organic cause, that is, sepsis or altered renal function.

History
It is important to rule out organic causes by exploring the history and physical symptoms with the patient, relatives and carers. Identify previous or current mental health history. Explore common features of hallucinations and delusions.

Hallucinations are false sensory perceptions that occur when the patient is awake. Examples include:

- Hearing voices (auditory) often telling the patient to carry out acts or self-harm
- Seeing objects (visual) that are not there – this can be indicative of an organic cause
- Feeling sensations on the skin (tactile)

Acute psychosis (continued)

Delusions are false beliefs that are often untrue. Common delusional features include:

- Persecutory – paranoia that a person or persons are attempting to harm them
- Jealousy – a strong sense of jealousy of others
- Grandiose – a belief centring around an over-inflated sense of self-worth
- Somatic – a strong belief that something is physically wrong with them
- Erotomanic – a belief that another person (often someone famous) is in love with them

Examination

Exclude underlying physical cause as appropriate with:

- Vital signs
- ECG
- Bloods
- CXR
- Urinalysis

Management

- Risk assess using mental health matrix and manage in appropriate clinical area according to local policies.
- Consider need for increased observations, 1:1 or RMN support to maintain safety.
- Exclude organic cause and if present initiate appropriate treatments.
- Where possible manage patient in a quiet area to reduce external stimulus.
- Refer to mental health services as per local protocols.

Acute anxiety and panic attacks

Definition

A panic attack is a sudden feeling of severe anxiety and fear sometimes without warning. The cause may be easily identified and relate to an existing fear or phobia, but panic attacks can also occur for no apparent reason.

History

Acute anxiety and panic attacks can present with a number of symptoms, and these can include one or more of the following:

- Palpitations
- Dry mouth
- Feeling that one is going to die or go mad
- Feeling hot or cold
- Sweating and trembling
- A feeling of being short of breath or choking
- Chest pain
- Nausea, dizziness or feeling faint
- Numbness and pins and needles particularly to hands and feet

Examination

Whilst the management is often based on careful history taking and the results of the clinical examination, it is important to exclude physical causes. The minimum specific assessment should include:

- Vital signs
- ECG

Further assessment may be required with bloods and a CXR if clinically appropriate to exclude or confirm a suspected physical cause.

Acute anxiety and panic attacks (continued)
Management

- Encourage patient to breathe as slowly and deeply as possible. Many patients concentrating on taking a long, slow breath in and then very slowly breathing out find that deep breathing exercises are useful. This means taking a long, slow breath in and then very slowly breathing out.
- Reassure the patient that the physical symptoms of a panic attack are not due to physical disease.
- No specific treatment is generally required if a patient has occasional panic attacks.
- Encourage the patient to discuss their symptoms with their GP if becoming regular or the patient is feeling consistently anxious.
- For patients who suffer with regular panic attacks, treatment is often required and includes cognitive behavioural therapy and the use of antidepressant medication.

Deliberate self-harm
Definition
Deliberate self-harm (DSH) covers a spectrum of self-inflicted injuries including cuts, burns, poisoning or asphyxiation.

History
Patients often have a history of DSH with an underlying mental health diagnosis. Many clinical settings have established management plans in place which detail support agencies engaged with the patient and advise regarding typical care required and follow-up/communication.

It is important to take a comprehensive history to ascertain any triggers for the episode of self-harm, the intention and how the patient feels following their action. It is important to build trust and ascertain the location of all injuries.

Examination and management
Wound care
- Examine, document and manage wounds as per general wound care guidance.
- Referral to appropriate specialties may be required if wounds involve underlying structures or are on the face.
- Ensure appropriate wound follow-up and removal of sutures if appropriate.

Foreign bodies
- Manage foreign bodies as per normal protocols.
- Referral to appropriate specialties may be required.

Attempted asphyxiation
- Manage as appropriate in line with ATLS protocols.
- Have a high index of suspicion for C-spine injuries in attempted hanging.

General principles
- Undertake mental health assessment matrix as per local guidance and procedures.
- Patients should be managed in an appropriate clinical area where direct observation is possible if unaccompanied or assessed as high risk.
- Consider the clinical environment and the risk of instruments, sharps, oxygen tubing, etc., that can lead to further attempts of self-harm.
- All patients will require appropriate follow-up either by already established support agencies on discharge or by the acute mental health team within the emergency or unscheduled care environment, depending on level of assessed risk.

Mental Health Act overview

Section 2	• Compulsory admission for assessment and treatment • 2 × doctors and approved mental health professional normally assess patient and make application • Can last up to 28 days
Section 3	• Compulsory admission for treatment • Same application procedure as for Section 2 • Can last up to 6 months and then reviewed
Section 4	• Emergency admission • Lasts initially for 72 hours • Similar application process as for Sections 2 and 3 but only one doctor is required
Section 136	• Applied by the police when they judge a person may harm themselves or others • Allows removal from public place to hospital for assessment • Not all Emergency Departments are considered a place of safety, and therefore assessment at a local mental health unit may be more appropriate

Note: Section 5 powers also exist under the Mental Health Act to prevent a patient leaving a hospital. This has not been included in the text as it is unlikely to apply to emergency and urgent care environments without a mental health practitioner being present to advise.

Musculoskeletal

Rapid Emergency and Unscheduled Care, First Edition. Oliver Phipps and Jason Lugg.
© 2016 John Wiley & Sons, Ltd. Published 2016 by John Wiley & Sons, Ltd.

Achilles tendon injuries

Definition

Achilles tendon rupture (partial or complete) refers to tearing of the Achilles tendon. The Achilles is the tendon that connects the calf muscles to the calcanium. Achilles tendinopathy (preferred term to tendonitis) is a broad term used to describe a degenerative condition that causes pain, swelling, weakness and stiffness of the Achilles tendon.

Aetiology

Achilles tendinopathy is believed to result from repeated micro trauma to the tendon that fails to heal. The mechanism of repeated tendon overloading causes degeneration. Achilles tendon rupture occurs when the tendon is overstretched. Rupture can be secondary to tendinopathy or occur in individuals who have suddenly increased their sporting activity.

Epidemiology

Achilles tendinopathy has an estimated lifetime incidence of around 6% in inactive people, but this increases to around 50% in elite athletes. Men are more likely to be affected particularly between 30 and 40 years of age. Achilles tendon rupture has an incidence of 6–18 ruptures per 100 000 people. Rupture is also more common in men, with complete rupture affecting three times more men than women.

History

- In tendinopathy the patient often describes a gradual onset of pain and swelling to the Achilles tendon with reduced range of movement due to stiffness. Pain is often in the middle third of the tendon and worse in the morning.
- In rupture the patient often describes a sudden and sometimes audible popping sensation to the back of the ankle (patients often initially think they were kicked), followed by pain, swelling and lack of function. Weight bearing can be difficult.

Examination

- Look for swelling or bruising along the tendon.
- Feel for the presence of a palpable gap or loss of contour indicating rupture.
- Assess active and resisted ankle plantar flexion.
- Perform a calf squeeze (Simmonds or Thompson test) and compare to the other leg.

Investigations

- Achilles tendinopathy is a clinical diagnosis, and imaging is not routinely required.
- X-ray is not usually of value unless suspecting other injuries, that is, calcanium avulsion.
- Ultrasound scanning or MRI is useful in secondary care to confirm diagnosis.

Management

Achilles tendinopathy	Achilles tendon rupture
• Advise rest in particular from high-impact activities • Inform patients symptoms can take 3–6 months to resolve • Cold packs are useful after acute injury • Analgesia (paracetamol or ibuprofen) • Refer to GP for ongoing management • Consider referral to physiotherapist	• Refer to emergency department • Place non-weight bearing in an equinus cast • Assess thromboembolism risk as per local protocol and refer if indicated • Refer to orthopaedic team as per local protocol. This normally involves referral to fracture clinic • Definitive management is either conservative or with surgical repair

Ankle injuries
Definition
Ankle injuries refer to fractures of the distal tibia or fibula, talus or calcanium. Injuries to the soft tissues of the ankle joint are also common presentations.

History
- Identify exact the mechanism of injury if possible.
- Weight bearing since (immediately, partially or not able to weight bear since injury).
- Previous injuries or problems with the ankle joint.
- Identify other injuries.
- First-aid measures undertaken.
- Analgesia taken.

Examination
Look
- Inspect for swelling, bruising, wounds, deformity and colour of the skin.

Feel
- Feel the skin temperature.
- Palpate and note the location of tenderness of the bones of the ankle and foot.
- Palpate and note the location of tenderness of the soft tissues.
- Palpate joints above and below.
- Palpate the fibula in ankle injuries.
- Check CRT, pulses and distal neurology.

Move
- If fracture suspected do not move joint.
- Otherwise assess ROM – inversion, eversion, plantar flexion and dorsiflexion.

Investigations
The Ottawa ankle rules provide a useful guide to the need for X-ray in ankle injuries and have a sensitivity of around 98% as follows:

- Tenderness to the posterior edge or tip of either malleolus along with the inability to weight bear immediately and at assessment indicates the need for an ankle X-ray.
- Tenderness localised over the navicular or base of the fifth metatarsal along with the inability to weight bear immediately or at assessment indicates the need for a foot X-ray.

Management

Injury or condition	Mechanism of injury	Clinical presentation	Treatment

Ankle fractures	Excessive inversion stress is the most common cause of ankle injuries. Eversion and rotational forces are other causes of fracture	• Swelling
		• Bruising
		• Deformity
		• Bony tenderness
		• Palpable fracture line
			• Management dependent on radiological and clinical findings
			• Refer patient to ED, MIU or appropriate urgent care setting according to local protocols
			• Simple and undisplaced:
			  ○ Immobilise in a below knee back slab*
			  ○ Non-weight bearing
			  ○ Refer to fracture clinic
			• Displaced fractures and bimalleolar, trimalleolar or intra-articular fractures:

Ankle injuries (continued)

Injury or condition	Mechanism of injury	Clinical presentation	Treatment
			o Refer to orthopaedics for guidance on management (These fractures often require open reduction and internal fixation (ORIF))
Ankle dislocation	Significant stress force with rotation and inversion. Concurrent fractures are common	• Obvious deformity • Swelling • Tenting of the skin	• Analgesia • Early reduction is essential • Reduce if adequate analgesia available and appropriately trained • Splint or plaster immediately • Refer to ED or directly to orthopaedics
Ankle sprain	Inversion or eversion of ankle joint	• Swelling • Bruising • Soft tissue tenderness	• **R**est ankle for 48–72 hours and consider supply of crutches • **I**ce – apply ice to ankle in a damp cloth for 15–20 minutes every 2–3 hours • **C**ompression – support with pillow (there is no strong evidence for compression bandaging in the acute phase) • **E**levation – raising the ankle above the heart will prevent and reduce swelling • Use simple analgesia as necessary • Advise patient to avoid heat, alcohol, running or massage (HARM) in the first 72 hours

*Placing patients that are non-weight bearing in below knee immobilisation is associated with increased risk of thromboembolism. Many centres now risk stratify for at-risk patients and provide appropriate prophylactic therapy.

Back pain (acute)
Definition
Lower back pain refers to pain in the lumbosacral area. Mechanical pack pain refers to the spinal joints and soft tissues; it varies with posture and is exacerbated by movement.

Aetiology
Lower back pain is often caused by heavy lifting or manual activity, although it is important to identify back pain caused by trauma, inflammatory disease or systemic illness. In inflammatory disease the pain often lasts longer than 30 minutes and is relieved by mobilising.

Epidemiology
It is estimated that lower back pain affects around one third of the UK adult population each year with around 20% consulting their GP.

History
• Identify mechanical cause if known.
• History of onset, duration, aggravation or relieving factors and treatment to date.
• Obtain a full past medical history.

Back pain (acute) (continued)

- Identify history of previous lower back pain.
- Ask about saddle anaesthesia or bladder or bowel dysfunction (indicates possible cauda equina syndrome).
- Analgesia taken.

Examination
Look
- Inspect for swelling, muscle spasm, bruising and deformity.

Feel
- Palpate central spinal processes for tenderness.
- Palpate paraspinal muscles for tenderness.
- Palpate across the back for tenderness and muscle spasm.

Move
- Assess ROM at the lumbar spine.
- Assess patient's ability to perform straight leg raise.

If abnormal neurology is suspected indicating nerve root pain, then assess lower limb sensation, power, tone and reflexes. If indicated, check saddle sensation and perform digital rectal examination to check anal tone.

Back pain red flags
- Presentation under 20 or onset over the age of 55
- Violent trauma
- Thoracic pain
- PMH of neoplasm
- Patient taking systemic steroids
- Constant, progressive non-mechanical pain
- Drug abuse or HIV
- Systemically unwell
- Weight loss
- Widespread neurological symptoms
- Bowel or bladder dysfunction

Investigations
Specific investigations are not required for simple uncomplicated back pain with no red flags. However if red flags are present or there is concern regarding the mechanism of injury, the patient will often require CT scan or MRI in the emergency or unscheduled care environment.

Management
- Reassure that most people with uncomplicated lower back pain make a good recovery.
- Advise regular analgesia with paracetamol with or without NSAID. If this is insufficient then consider weak opioid.
- If significant muscle spasm consider short course of muscle relaxant.
- Encourage early physical activity.
- Advise follow-up with patient's GP if symptoms continue for 4–6 weeks.
- Advise patient of red flag symptoms and the need to seek urgent medical review.

Calcanium fractures

Definition
Calcanium fractures refer to fracture of the calcanium or heel bone.

Aetiology
Axial loading is the normal mechanism of injury, although calcanium stress fractures can also occur. Jumping from a height is a common presentation.

History
- Identify the mechanism of injury if possible.
- Weight bearing since (immediately, partially or not able to weight bear since injury).
- Identify other injuries (spinal and pelvic injuries can also occur with axial loading mechanism).
- First-aid measures undertaken.
- Analgesia taken.

Examination
Look
- Inspect for swelling, bruising and wounds.

Feel
- Palpate and note the location of tenderness of the bones of the ankle and foot.
- Palpate and note the location of tenderness of the soft tissues.
- Assess for spinal, pelvic and other lower limb injuries.
- Check CRT, pulses and distal neurology.

Move
- Assess ROM if no injury suspected at ankle, knee and hip joints to help exclude other injuries.

Investigations
- X-ray with calcanium views (lateral view essential to calculate Bohler's angle $\leq 20°$ indicates fracture).
- Other X-rays will also be required if other injuries are suspected.
- MRI and CT scan are also routinely performed to visualise extent of fracture.

Management
- Non-weight bearing immediately with crutches.
- Below knee back slab plaster.
- Elevation to reduce swelling.
- Refer to fracture clinic or discuss with orthopaedic surgeons according to local protocols.

Compartment syndrome

Definition
Acute compartment syndrome relates to local tissue ischaemia and hypoxia due to raised pressure within the fascial compartment.

Aetiology
Most cases of compartment syndrome are seen following fractures and crush injuries. Restrictive dressings and casts can also cause the syndrome. The raised pressure within the closed fascial compartment leads to ischaemia and hypoxia. Prompt diagnosis and intervention are vital to avoid severe disability.

Compartment syndrome (continued)
History
- Careful history of events leading up to symptoms (recent injury and treatments).
- Careful pain history – pain in compartment syndrome is normally disproportionate to what would reasonably be expected for the injury.
- Assess other symptoms, that is, altered neurology.
- Analgesia taken and effect.

Examination
Look
- Inspect and compare both limbs for swelling, bruising, wounds, deformity and colour of the skin.

Feel
- Feel the skin temperature.
- Palpate the limb carefully noting location of tenderness.
- Check CRT, pulses and distal neurology.

Move
- Assess movement of joint above and below the suspected compartment.

> **TOP TIP:**
> - Distal pulses are often present in compartment syndrome
> - Regional anaesthesia, altered level of consciousness or opiate analgesia can mask symptoms

Investigations
- Compartment syndrome is initially a clinical diagnosis.
- Compartment pressures are recorded. A compartment pressure >40 mmHg to the diastolic pressure is an absolute diagnosis of compartment syndrome.

Management
- Compartment syndrome is a SURGICAL EMERGENCY.
- Urgent referral to orthopaedics is required.
- Decompression of the fascial compartment by fasciotomies is indicated and ideally should be performed within an hour of the decision to operate.

Elbow injuries
Definition
Elbow injuries and conditions cover a range of presentations including:

- Supracondylar humeral fractures – fracture to the distal humerus above the epicondyles.
- Dislocated elbow.
- Olecranon bursitis – inflammation of the olecranon bursa (can be inflammatory or septic).
- Epicondylitis – tendinopathy by repeated micro trauma. Injuries can involve the lateral extensor tendon (tennis elbow) or the medial flexor tendon (golfers elbow).
- Radial head fractures – fractures to the radial head are often occult injuries.

History
- Identify the exact mechanism of injury.
- Identify function since injury or symptoms.

Elbow injuries (continued)

- Enquire about possible causes of tendinopathy.
- Previous injuries or problems with the elbow joint.
- Identify other possible injuries.
- First-aid measures undertaken.
- Analgesia taken.

Examination

Look
- Inspect for swelling, bruising, wounds, deformity and colour of the skin.

Feel
- Feel the skin temperature.
- Palpate and note the location of tenderness of the bones of the elbow.
- Palpate and note the location of tenderness of the soft tissues.
- Palpate the humerus, ulna, radius and wrist and shoulder joints.

Move
- If fracture suspected do not move joint.
- Otherwise assess ROM – flexion, extension, supination and pronation.

Investigations
- Elbow X-ray is the most common method of imaging and is indicated when the mechanism of injury and clinical examination suggest bony injury. X-ray is not routinely indicated in suspected soft tissue injuries.

Management
Specific elbow injuries are discussed as follows:

Injury or condition	Mechanism of injury	Clinical presentation	Treatment
Supracondylar humeral fractures	Supracondylar fractures represent most common elbow fracture in children with a peak age between 5 and 8 years. The usual mechanism is a fall onto the outstretched hand with hyperextension at the elbow	• Swelling • Bruising • Deformity to the elbow • Bony tenderness to distal humerus • May have distal neurovascular compromise (red flag)	• Analgesia • Above elbow back slab • Referral to orthopaedics Displaced fractures require immediate referral to orthopaedics
Dislocated elbow	Elbow dislocations are not common injuries. The usual mechanism for elbow dislocation is a fall on an outstretched hand. It is the force transmitted to the elbow, often with a rotational action that can dislocate the joint	• Extreme elbow pain • Obvious deformity • Lower arm may look rotated • May have distal neurovascular compromise (red flag)	• Analgesia • Refer to ED for immediate reduction • Above elbow back slab • Referral to orthopaedics

(Continued)

Injury or condition	Mechanism of injury	Clinical presentation	Treatment
Olecranon bursitis	The usual mechanism is overuse or mild trauma (e.g. leaning on elbow) that can cause the condition. Systemic conditions (gout, rheumatoid arthritis, systemic lupus, ankylosing spondylitis) can increase incidence of bursitis	• Swelling over the olecranon process that has appeared over hours or days • Swelling is warm, tender and fluctuant in nature • Elbow range of movement is normal apart from full flexion	• Rest, apply ice and reduce activity • Compressive bandaging (elasticated tubular bandage may be helpful if tolerated) • Analgesia – paracetamol or NSAID • Advise the need to avoid/minimise trauma to the elbow • Reassure that most people will respond to conservative treatment • Advise seeking medical review if symptoms appear to be worsening • Refer to GP for ongoing management
	Septic bursitis occurs when bacteria enter the bursa (olecranon bursae are more susceptible due to its superficial nature)	Consider septic bursitis when: • Painful, red and hot swelling of the bursa which has progressed over last few days • Evidence of local cellulitis • Abrasion or laceration over the bursa • Fever	
		(Suspect another diagnosis if there is generalised joint swelling)	If septic bursitis is suspected: • Treat with oral antibiotic as per local guidelines • GP review in 7 days
Epicondylitis	Repetitive, forceful work or leisure activity often causes the tendon swelling	*Tennis elbow:*	
	In tennis elbow mechanisms include repetitive heavy lifting or the use of heavy tools and new and unaccustomed strains to the elbow joint	• Gradual onset • Pain and tenderness of the lateral epicondyle (commonly in the dominant arm) • Pain may radiate into the forearm • Increased pain on resisted dorsiflexion of the wrist • Normal elbow range of movement	• Avoid reducing identified cause of symptoms • Advise NSAIDs if not contraindicated with paracetamol with or without codeine • Consider topical NSAIDs or gastroprotection if adverse effects are likely • If symptoms persist refer to GP for ongoing management (may benefit from corticosteroid infection or referral to physiotherapy)
	In golfers elbow mechanisms include sports involving gripping or throwing and new jobs or hobbies that require repetitive elbow movements	*Golfers elbow:* • Pain and tenderness over the medial epicondyle • Pain may radiate to the forearm • Increased pain on wrist flexion and pronation	

Elbow injuries (continued)

Injury or condition	Mechanism of injury	Clinical presentation	Treatment
		• Gradual onset of pain and discomfort • An associated neuropathy may be present and cause altered sensation in the ring and little fingers	
Radial head fracture	Fractured radial heads (20% of all elbow fractures) usually occur from a fall on an outstretched hand. It is the force transmitted to the elbow that can lead to a radial head fracture	• Pain and swelling to the elbow • Tenderness to the radial head • Stiff and general painful joint on movement • Unable to fully extend the elbow • Painful supination and pronation This is often an occult fracture and not easily seen on X-ray. Elevated fat pads are the classic sign indicating a fracture	• Analgesia • Refer to local protocols, often broad arm sling • Referral to fracture clinic If displaced or distal neurovascular compromise, then refer for immediate orthopaedic assessment

Femoral injuries
Definition
Femoral fractures are commonly divided into three anatomical categories, proximal, mid-shaft and distal. Fractures of the neck of femur are common in the elderly and occur often after falls and are increased in the presence of osteoporosis. Mid-shaft and distal femur fractures are commonly caused by high-impact trauma mechanism.

> **Important point:**
> Mid-shaft and distal femoral fractures indicate high-energy trauma. The injuries can be associated with significant hypovolaemia due to internal blood loss. Consider the need to manage as major trauma and initiate local arrangements as necessary

History
- Identify the exact mechanism of injury if possible.
- In cases related to falls careful history taking is important to ascertain the cause of fall and rule out collapse.
- Weight bearing since (immediately, partially or not able to weight bear since injury).
- Previous injuries or problems with the hip joint.
- Past medical history (e.g. osteoporosis).
- Identify other injuries.
- First-aid measures undertaken.
- Analgesia taken.

Femoral injuries (continued)
Examination
Vital signs (RR, HR, BP, temp, CRT and SpO_2) to assess haemodynamic status and assist in identifying causes of falls in the elderly

Look
- Inspect the entire leg for swelling, bruising, wounds, deformity and colour of the skin.
- Look for internal and external rotation of the leg.

Feel
- Feel the skin temperature.
- Palpate and note the location of tenderness of the pelvis, hip, femur and knee.
- Palpate and note the location of tenderness of the soft tissues.
- Check CRT, pulses and distal neurology.

Move
- If fracture suspected do not move joint until excluded.
- Otherwise assess ROM:
  Hip – flexion, extension, internal and external rotation, abduction, adduction and straight leg raise
  Knee – flexion and extension
- Assess weight bearing and gait.

Investigations
- Select appropriate plain film X-ray for provisional diagnosis following history and examination which may include pelvis, hip, femur and knee views.
- In major trauma CT scan is often the initial source of imaging.
- Bloods (FBC, U&Es, LFTs, TFTs and clotting screen). Group and save with or without crossmatching if there is concern regarding hypovolaemia.
- ECG if arrhythmia is suspected as the cause for fall.

Management
- Manage as ABCDE approach if major trauma.
- Prehospital – 999 ambulance to ED.
- ED management should involve early assistance from orthopaedic team.

Injury or condition	Mechanism of injury	Clinical presentation	Treatment

Neck of femur fractures	Most common in the elderly following a fall. In younger patients the mechanism usually involves high-energy impact	• Bruising and swelling around the hip
		• Deformity – shortening and external rotation of the leg
		• Unable to do straight leg raise or actively move the hip
			• Analgesia
			• Prehospital – 999 ambulance to ED
			• Most hospitals have specific care pathways for the management of the neck of femur fractures. These include:
			  ○ Adequate analgesia including regional anaesthesia
			  ○ Referral to orthopaedics for admission to inpatient bed
			  ○ IV fluids as required

Femoral injuries (continued)

Injury or condition	Mechanism of injury	Clinical presentation	Treatment
Mid-shaft fractures	Normally a high-energy injury (RTC). Pathological fractures can occur in osteoporotic or patients with metastatic disease	• Swelling • Bruising • Deformity to the femur	• Prehospital – 999 ambulance to ED • ABCDE approach • IV access and bloods • IV fluids as indicated • Traction to femur • Analgesia • Referral to orthopaedic team
	Often associated with injuries to the hip, pelvis and knee		(Blood loss can result by 1000–1500 ml in femoral shaft fractures. It is important to manage signs of hypovolaemic shock)
Supracondylar fractures	Normally a high-energy injury (RTC). Pathological fractures can occur in osteoporotic or patients with metastatic disease	• Pain more focused around the knee • Swelling and bruising to the distal femur and knee	• Analgesia • Prehospital – 999 ambulance to ED • Refer to orthopaedic team (treatment dependent on fracture classification and displacement – managed either conservatively in plaster/knee brace or by surgery)

Foot injuries
Definition
Foot fractures account for around 10% of all fractures. They can be severe injuries with the potential to cause long-term pain and loss of function. Outcome is worse where there is a delay in appropriate treatment. Stress fractures to the foot occur in athletes.

History
- Identify the exact mechanism of injury if possible.
- Weight bearing since (immediately, partially or not able to weight bear since injury).
- Previous injuries or problems with the foot.
- Past medical history (e.g. osteoporosis).
- Identify other injuries.
- First-aid measures undertaken.
- Analgesia taken.

Examination
Look
- Inspect for swelling, bruising, wounds, deformity and colour of the skin.

Feel
- Feel the skin temperature.
- Palpate and note the location of tenderness of the bones of the foot and ankle.
- Palpate and note the location of tenderness of the soft tissues and plantar surface.
- Check CRT, pulses and distal neurology.

Move
- If fracture suspected do not move ankle or toes until excluded.
- Otherwise assess ROM at the ankle.
- Assess ability to weight bear if fracture is excluded.

Foot injuries (continued)
Investigations
• If bony injury suspected request and evaluate foot films (normally AP and oblique).

Management

Injury or condition	Mechanism of injury	Clinical presentation	Treatment
Tarsal bone fractures (talus, navicular, cuboid, medial, intermediate and lateral cuneiforms) Calcanium fractures are covered separately in this section	Tarsal bone fractures occur due to direct trauma, awkwardly landing on the foot from jumping and/or twisting injury. Talus fractures can be caused by excessive dorsiflexion at the ankle with axial load. Stress fractures can occur to the navicular and calcanium bones	• Bruising and swelling to foot • Specific point tenderness to one or more tarsal bones	• Analgesia • Non-weight bearing • Below knee POP or walking boot dependent on local protocols* • Crutches • Referral to fracture clinic
Metatarsal fractures	The most common mechanism occurs when the forefoot is fixed and the hindfoot is rotated. Crush injury is another cause Avulsion of the base of the fifth metatarsal can occur following inversion injury	• Swelling • Bruising • Focal or diffuse area of tenderness • Inability to weight bear	• Analgesia • Non-weight bearing • Below knee POP or walking boot dependent on local protocols* • Crutches • Referral to fracture clinic
Toe fractures	Normally caused by direct trauma (dropping an object directly onto toe) or stubbing toe on an object	• Bruising • Swelling • Redness • Wounds • Sometimes deformity X-ray is only indicated for great toes or when there is suspected dislocation or displaced fractures	Simple fractures to small toes: • Analgesia • Neighbour strapping • Advise patient to wear comfortable shoes • No follow-up required and should have settled in 4–6 weeks Dislocation/displacement: • Analgesia • Local anaesthetic/nerve block or Entonox® • Relocate or realign • Immobilise or splint • Check X-ray • Recheck neurovascular status • Refer to local protocols whether follow-up is required The great toe is treated as above, but normal practice is to refer to fracture clinic

*Placing patients that are non-weight bearing in below knee immobilisation is associated with increased risk of thromboembolism. Many centres now risk stratify for at-risk patients and provide appropriate prophylactic therapy.

Foot injuries (continued)

Lisfranc injuries
Lisfranc injuries represent serious ligamental injuries and can cause significant disruption to the tarsometatarsal joint. It is easily missed and mistaken for a soft tissue injury, and X-ray findings can be very subtle. The mechanism is often a low-energy twisting action or a forced downward flexion at the mid-foot. Specific signs that should increase your suspicion of Lisfranc injury include:
- Significant swelling and pain to the dorsum of the foot
- Bruising to the plantar surface of the foot
- Pain disproportionate to the clinical suspicion

Gastrocnemius muscle tears
Definition
Gastrocnemius muscle tears refer to the tearing of the muscle fibres of the gastrocnemius (calf) muscle.

Aetiology
It is most commonly seen in middle-aged recreational athletes. The mechanism involves sudden force on the muscle greater than the permitted tension. Specific actions that can lead to a gastrocnemius tear include activity that requires a sudden change in direction (e.g. hill running, tennis and basketball).

History
- Identify the exact mechanism of injury if possible.
- Weight bearing since (immediately, partially or not able to weight bear since injury).
- Previous injuries or problems with the calf.
- First-aid measures undertaken.
- Analgesia taken.

Examination
Look
- Inspect and compare both limbs for swelling, bruising and colour of the skin.

Feel
- Palpate the muscle body and Achilles tendon.
- Palpate the limb carefully noting the location of tenderness.
- Check CRT, pulses and distal neurology.

Move
- Exclude Achilles tendon rupture by performing calf squeeze test.
- Assess ROM at the knee and ankle joint.

> **TOP TIP:**
> Achilles tendon rupture occurs in a similar mechanism; it is therefore important to exclude Achilles rupture before diagnosing a gastrocnemius tear. Refer to Achilles tendon rupture earlier in this section.
> Deep vein thrombosis is a differential diagnosis in a patient with gastrocnemius tear.

Investigations
- Gastrocnemius tear is a clinical diagnosis, and routine investigations are not usually required.
- Ultrasound imaging or MRI may be indicated if there is concern regarding Achilles tendon rupture.

Gastrocnemius muscle tears (continued)
Management
- Rest, apply ice and reduce activity.
- Crutches may be required for short-term use only.
- Analgesia – paracetamol or NSAID.
- Reassure that most people respond well to conservative treatment in around 2 weeks.
- Footwear with a slightly raised heal can provide relief in symptoms.
- Advise seeking GP review if symptoms appear to be getting worse or not resolving.

Hand injuries
Definition
Hand injuries cover a range of soft tissue and bony injuries. These include fractures to the metacarpals, fingers and thumb and common tendon injuries such as mallet and boutonniere deformities. Hand injuries are common presentations, and methodical assessment is essential in identifying the extent of damage to structures of the hand, which are easily overlooked and can cause long-term functional problems.

History
- Identify the exact mechanism and time of injury.
- Identify function since injury or symptoms.
- Previous injuries or problems with hands.
- First-aid measures undertaken.
- Analgesia taken.
- Hand dominance.
- Occupation and relevant recreational hobbies.

Examination
Look
- Inspect for swelling, bruising, wounds, deformity and colour of the skin.
- Look for finger lag in finger injuries.

Feel
- Feel the skin temperature and check CRT in the fingers and thumb.
- Palpate and note the location of tenderness of the bones of the hand.
- Palpate and note the location of tenderness of the soft tissues.
- Check the sensation and motor function carefully of the radial, medial and ulnar nerves.
- Examine the wrist for signs of injury.

Move
- If fracture suspected do not move joint.
- Check active, passive and resisted movement of the key tendons of the thumb and fingers.
- Check for rotational deformity in suspected fractures of the fifth metacarpal.
- Check ROM at the wrist (flexion, extension, ulnar and radial deviation).

Investigations
- X-ray is an essential tool in diagnosing hand injuries. Views include hand films (PA and oblique). Specific thumb and finger views are valuable for specific injury locations. Crush injuries should always be X-rayed to identify fractures.

Management
- Analgesia.
- Remove all rings early.
- Elevate early to minimise swelling and aid examination.

Hand injuries (continued)

Specific hand injuries are discussed as follows:

Injury or condition	Mechanism of injury	Clinical presentation	Treatment
Fracture of the base of the first metacarpal – Bennett's fractures (often associated with subluxation)	Axial loading with a partially flexed thumb	• Swelling and bruising to the base of the thumb and thenar eminence • Tenderness to the thumb metacarpal base • Reduced range of movement and instability at the CMC joint	Undisplaced: • Bennett's POP • High arm sling • Referral to fracture clinic Displaced: • High arm sling • Referral to orthopaedics/plastic/hand surgeons dependent on local protocols
Fracture of the fourth or fifth metacarpal head (Boxer's fracture)	Caused by a punch to a hard object with closed fist	• Pain and tenderness localised to the metacarpal head • Bruising and swelling to the metacarpal head, often with associated wounds • Rotation of the little finger can be present when asked to make a fist	• Volar slab or neighbour strapping dependent on swelling and pain + refer to local protocols • High arm sling • Referral to orthopaedics/plastic/hand surgeons dependent on local protocols Discuss very displaced fractures with appropriate surgical specialty as above prior to discharge
Metacarpal fractures	Direct blow to the hand or rotational injury with axial load	• Pain and tenderness • Bruising and swelling • Explore wounds carefully as may reveal open fracture or damage to deeper structures. Dorsal wounds can affect the sensory branch of the radial/medial and ulnar nerves. Volar wounds can involve the digital nerves	• Below elbow POP with MCP joints in 70–90° of flexion (refer to local protocols) • High arm sling • Referral to orthopaedics/plastic/hand surgeons dependent on local protocols Discuss very displaced fractures with appropriate surgical specialty as above prior to discharge
Ulnar collateral ligament rupture (often referred to as skier's thumb or gamekeeper's thumb)	Fall onto the outstretched thumb. The injury is more likely if the thumb is gripping something at the same time. Hyperextension and abduction can also cause the injury	• Pain and tenderness to the base of the thumb and metacarpal – carpal joint • Swelling and bruising • Inability to grip or hold objects firmly	• Thumb spica • Elevation as swelling dictates • Referral to orthopaedics/plastic/hand surgeons dependent on local protocols

(Continued)

Hand injuries (continued)

Injury or condition	Mechanism of injury	Clinical presentation	Treatment
	Injury can be ligament only or associated with avulsion fracture of the proximal phalanx	• Pain and/or laxity on gentle stressing UCL (compare to the other thumb) • Sometime a swelling can be palpated to the ulnar side of the base of the thumb	
Proximal and middle phalanx fractures	Mechanism for finger fractures include crush injuries, blunt force, rotation and secondary to lacerations from power tools. Avulsion fractures can occur when fingers are hyperextended	• Localised finger tenderness to the affected phalanx • Swelling and bruising • Wounds may be present • Reduced range of movement at PIPJ/DIPJ	• Analgesia • Neighbour strapping • High arm sling • Referral to fracture clinic
Distal phalanx fractures		Subungual haematoma may be present with distal phalanx fractures	• Analgesia • Consider neighbour strapping for comfort (not clinically indicated) • Trephining subungual haematoma if present • High arm sling • Referral to fracture clinic
Mallet deformity	Telescoping or object hitting tip of finger causing forced flexion at the DIPJ – causing extensor tendon rupture with or without avulsion fracture	• Painful and swollen DIPJ • Evident distal phalanx droop at DIPJ • Able to flex at DIPJ but no active distal phalanx extension	• Immobilise in mallet or Zimmer splint • Careful instructions need to be given to patient around self-care management • Referral to hand physiotherapy as per local protocols • Referral to orthopaedics/plastics/hand surgeons if avulsion fracture present as per local protocols
Boutonniere deformity	Occurs when a finger PIPJ is flexed at the same time as the DIPJ is extended. The usual cause is a stubbing injury	• Pain and swelling of the PIPJ • Finger is fixed in flexion at PIPJ • Unable to actively extend finger at PIPJ • Unable to flex finger at DIPJ	• Neighbour strap • High arm sling • Referral to orthopaedics/plastics/hand surgeons as per local protocols

Knee injuries
Definition
Knee injuries cover a range of soft tissue and bony injuries. These include fractured and dislocation of the patella, injuries to the cruciate and collateral ligaments and menisci injuries. Knee injuries are common presentations in emergency and unscheduled care settings and are often difficult to comprehensively assess in the acute phase due to pain and swelling.

History
- Identify the exact mechanism and time of injury (direct force, twisting, valgus or varus strain, was the patient weight bearing at time of injury?).
- Does the knee give way or lock?
- Identify function since injury – able to fully or partially weight bear immediately or progressively deteriorated.
- Enquire onset of swelling (rapid < 2 hours or more gradual).
- Previous injuries or problems with knees.
- First-aid measures undertaken.
- Analgesia taken.
- Occupation and relevant recreational hobbies.

Examination
Look
- Assess weight bearing and gait.
- Inspect for swelling/effusion, bruising, wounds, deformity and colour of the skin.

Feel
- Feel the skin temperature.
- Palpate and note the location of the bony tenderness to:
  Distal femur and femoral condyles
  Patella
  Medical and lateral joint line
  Medical and lateral tibial plateau
  Fibular head
  Popliteal fossa
- Palpate and note any gap or contour loss to quadriceps and patella.
- Check sensation distally, along with peripheral pulses and CRT.
- Check for joint effusion with bulge test.

Move
- If fracture suspected do not move joint until excluded.
- Assess ability to perform straight leg raise.
- Check active and passive movement of joint (flexion and extension).
- Perform valgus and varus stress tests for pain and laxity to collateral ligaments.
- Perform anterior draw or Lachman's test to assess anterior cruciate ligament.
- Perform posterior draw test of posterior sag test for posterior cruciate ligament.
- Assess ROM at the hip and ankle joint.

It is essential to examine the uninjured knee to make an accurate comparison.

Investigations
The Ottawa knee rules provide a useful guide to the need for X-ray in emergency and unscheduled care settings. The following indicate the need for a knee X-ray:

- Age > 55 years
- Isolated patella tenderness

Knee injuries (continued)

- Tenderness to the fibular head
- Unable to flex to 90°
- Inability to weight bear both immediately and during consultations for four steps

In suspected patella fractures make sure specific patella views are requested.

Management

- Analgesia

Specific knee injuries are discussed as follows:

Injury or condition	Mechanism of injury	Clinical presentation	Treatment
Anterior cruciate ligament injury	• Sudden deceleration, stopping or changing direction with fixed foot • Hyperextension of the knee	• Swelling acute in onset • Reduced range of movement • Positive anterior draw or Lachman's test	• Rest • Apply ice • Elevate • Advise regular simple analgesia • Crutches as required • Refer as per local protocols (fracture or physiotherapy clinic) for review when injury less acute
Posterior cruciate ligament injury	• Direct blow to proximal tibia with knee in flexion (e.g. fall on flexed knee or RTC knee striking dashboard) • Hyperextension of knee	• Swelling • Reduced range of movement • Positive posterior draw or sag test • May present posterior knee pain	
Medical collateral ligament injury	• Direct blow to lateral aspect of knee, twisting or valgus strain	• Pain and tenderness along the MCL • Swelling acute in onset • Increased pain with or without laxity on valgus stress testing *(MCL injury is often accompanied with cruciate and meniscus injuries)*	• Rest • Apply ice • Elevate • Advise regular simple analgesia • Knee braces are often applied (refer to local protocols) • Crutches as required • Refer as per local protocols (fracture or physiotherapy clinic) for review when injury less acute
Lateral collateral ligament injury	• Direct blow to medical aspect of knee or varus strain	• Pain and tenderness along LCL • Swelling • Increased pain with or without laxity on varus stressing	• Rest • Apply ice • Elevate • Advise regular simple analgesia • Crutches as required • Refer as per local protocols (fracture or physiotherapy clinic) for review when injury less acute

Injury or condition	Mechanism of injury	Clinical presentation	Treatment
Patella fracture	• Direct blow to the patella as the most common mechanism	• Pain • Swelling with or without effusion • Extension block • X-ray findings (beware the bipartite patella)	• Analgesia • Non-weight bearing and crutches • Immobilise in POP or knee brace dependent on local protocols • Refer to fracture clinic • Discuss with orthopaedic team if significant displacement
Dislocated patella	• Direct blow to the medial aspect of the knee • History of dislocation and subsequent reduction	• Obvious lateral deformity if still dislocated • Painful and swollen medial aspect of the knee • Swelling • Reluctance to weight bear	• Reduce if still dislocated by extension with analgesia and if required muscle relaxant • X-ray to exclude fracture and presence of haemarthrosis • Immobilise in knee splint • Refer as per local protocols (fracture or physiotherapy clinic)
Meniscus injury	• Twisting or pivoting of the knee with minimal force required • Often weight bearing at time of injury	• Swelling gradual in onset • Joint line pain on the injured side • May complain of locking, catching or knee giving way	• Rest • Apply ice • Elevate • Advise regular simple analgesia • Crutches may be required during acute stage • Refer as per local protocols (fracture or physiotherapy clinic)
Pre-patella bursitis	• Repetitive friction to the bursa often by direct pressure. Common in individuals who use the kneel regularly • Systemic conditions (rheumatoid arthritis) can increase incidence of bursitis • Septic bursitis occurs when bacteria enter the bursa	• Rapid, localised and fluctuant swelling over the front of the patella • Tender and warm to palpation • Pain increases with activity and on flexion	• Rest, apply ice and reduce activity • Analgesia – paracetamol or NSAID • Reassure that most people will respond to conservative treatment • Advise seeking medical review if symptoms appear to be getting worse • Refer to GP for ongoing management
		Consider septic bursitis when: • Painful, red and hot swelling of the bursa • Evidence of local cellulitis • Abrasion or laceration over the bursa • Fever	If septic bursitis is suspected: • Treat with oral antibiotic as per local guidelines • GP review in 7 days and give guidance on when to seek earlier review

Neck pain: Traumatic neck sprain
Definition
Sudden movement of the head in any direction can cause a traumatic neck sprain (avoid the term whiplash). Traumatic neck sprain refers to a soft tissue injury to the neck.

Aetiology
Forced hyperextension and then flexion is the common mechanism. Rear-end shunt RTCs are very common presentation.

History
- Identify the mechanism of injury, speed of impact and whether seat belt was being worn.
- History of onset, duration, aggravation or relieving factors and treatment to date.
- Enquire about upper limb neurology.
- Obtain a full past medical history.
- Analgesia taken.

Examination
Look
- Inspect neck and shoulders for swelling, muscle spasm, bruising and deformity.

Feel
- Palpate central spinal processes for tenderness.
- Palpate paraspinal muscles for tenderness.
- Palpate shoulders for tenderness and muscle spasm.
- Check upper limb neurovascular status.

Move
- Do not move neck if red flags are suspected spinal injury.
- Assess ROM at C-spine.
- Assess ROM for both shoulders.

If abnormal neurology or red flag is present, then consider C-spine immobilisation.

Neck pain red flags
- Significant mechanism of injury
- Tenderness over spinal process
- Severe pain
- Neurological signs and symptoms

Investigations
Specific investigations are not required for simple uncomplicated neck pain with no red flags. However, if red flags are present or there is concern regarding the mechanism of injury, the patient will often require C-spine X-rays, CT imaging or MRI in the emergency or unscheduled care environment.

Management
- Advise regular analgesia with paracetamol with or without NSAID. If this is insufficient then consider weak opioid.
- If there is significant muscle spasm, consider short course of muscle relaxant.
- Encourage normal physical activity.
- If possible provide patient information leaflet on self-care management.
- Advise follow-up with patients GP if symptoms are getting worse or not settling in 2 weeks.

Pelvic fractures

Fractures to the pelvis are serious injuries and are orthopaedic emergencies. Major blood loss can cause life-threatening hypovolaemia.

Aetiology

High-energy forces cause most pelvic fractures. Falls from a significant height with axial loading, RTCs and crush injuries are common examples. Pelvic fractures can also occur in individuals with osteoporosis and can occur from simple falls from standing.

History

- Identify the mechanism of injury if possible.
- Identify other injuries (spinal and calcanium and lower limb injuries can also occur in axial loading mechanism).
- Prehospital interventions.
- Analgesia administered.

Examination

Symptoms

- Severe pelvic pain
- Swelling and bruising to the pelvis
- Swelling and bruising to the scrotum
- Pain to flank and perianal region

Signs

- Leg length and rotation of the limb without limb fracture.
- Signs of shock.
- Patient may benefit from positioning with knees slightly flexed.
- Blood at the urethra indicated urethral injury.
- Swollen testicles indicating possible testicular rupture.
- Absent or reduced femoral pulses.
- Rectal bleeding.
- Reduced anal tone on digital rectal examination suggests sacral spine involvement.

Investigations

- Bloods (FBC, U&Es, LFTs, TFTs and clotting screen; group and save and crossmatching).
- In major trauma CT scan is often the initial source of imaging.
- Other X-rays will also be required if other injuries are suspected.

Management

- Manage as ABCDE approach if major trauma.
- Prehospital – 999 ambulance to ED.
- IV access and bloods.
- Fluid management in line with latest trauma guidelines.
- Analgesia.
- Pelvic splint.
- Nil by mouth.
- Refer to orthopaedic team.

Plantar fasciitis

Definition

Plantar fasciitis is a condition in which there is persistent pain associated with inflammation and chronic degeneration to the plantar fascia.

Plantar fasciitis (continued)

Aetiology
Axial loading is the normal mechanism of injury for a fractured calcanium, although calcanium stress fractures do also occur. Jumping from a height is a common presentation.

History
- Onset of heel pain
- Intense pain during the first steps after waking or after a period of inactivity
- Pain worsens later during the day or after long periods of standing or walking

Examination
- Tenderness to the plantar heel area localised around the medial calcaneal tuberosity.
- Reduced ankle dorsiflexion with the knee in extension.
- Abnormal walking/limping due to pain may be observed.

Investigations
- Plantar fasciitis is a clinical diagnosis, and no specific investigations are initially useful.

Management
- Advise rest of the foot and avoid standing or walking for long periods.
- Wear shoes with adequate arch support.
- Analgesia as required – paracetamol and NSAIDs.
- Local application of an ice pack can provide symptomatic relief.
- Refer to GP for ongoing management if not settling – physiotherapy, podiatry or orthotics can provide useful interventions. Occasionally corticosteroid injections are indicated.

Pulled elbow

Definition
Pulled elbow refers to radial head subluxation. It is a minor soft tissue injury affecting children under 6 years of age, with a with peak incidence around 2–3 years.

Aetiology
Pulled elbow typically occurs following an axial pull on a child's arm (swinging a child in play or pulling a child back by their arm). It occurs when the radial head slips from the annular ligament.

History and symptoms
- Age and history suggest diagnosis.
- No history of trauma.
- Elbow pain and not moving the affected arm at elbow.
- Elbow often held slightly flexed and pronated.
- Swelling and tenderness to the radial head.

Investigations
- Pulled elbow is a clinical diagnosis based on history and clinical examination. X-ray is not indicated unless suspicion of other injuries exists or reduction is unsuccessful after two to three attempts.

Management
- Analgesia.
- Reduction if competent and experienced. Two main techniques include:
  - Flexion and forced supination while gently pressing on the radial head
  - Hyperpronation while pressing on the radial head
- Observe child until they start using the arm again (up to 1 hour).

Pulled elbow (continued)

- Arm sling if required.
- No formal follow-up required.
- There is a risk of recurrent injury; therefore explanation to parents of preventative measures should be provided.

Shoulder and clavicle injuries

Shoulder and clavicle injuries include a range of presentations including clavicle fractures, shoulder dislocations, acromioclavicular joint (ACJ) injury and soft tissue injuries.

History

- Identify the exact mechanism of injury if known.
- Identify shoulder function since injury or symptoms.
- Previous injuries or problems with the shoulder joint.
- First-aid measures undertaken.
- Analgesia taken.
- Hand dominance.
- Occupation and recreational hobbies.

Examination

Look

- Inspect for symmetry, swelling, bruising, wounds, deformity, muscles spasm and colour of the skin.

Feel

- Feel the skin temperature.
- Palpate the humerus, scapula, acromion, ACJ, coracoid and clavicle and note for tenderness.
- Palpate and note the location of tenderness of the soft tissues of the shoulder and neck.
- Examine C-spine and elbow joints for injury.
- Test distal neurovascular status.

Move

- Observe ROM initially when patient undresses.
- If fracture suspected do not move joint.
- Otherwise assess ROM – abduction, adduction, flexion, extension and internal and external rotation.
- Assess ROM at elbow and C-spine.

Investigations

- Shoulder X-ray is indicated if there is suspected fracture or dislocation. Specific clavicle and ACJ views should be requested if injury is suspected.

Management

Specific shoulder injuries are discussed as follows:

Injury or condition	Mechanism of injury	Clinical presentation	Treatment
Clavicle fractures	Direct blow to the shoulder or fall on an outstretched arm	• Swelling and bruising • Tender palpable deformity to the clavicle • Decreased range of movement with crepitus on movement • Check for skin tenting	• Broad arm sling • Analgesia • Refer to fracture clinic • Discuss with orthopaedic team if skin tenting or significant displacement

(Continued)

Shoulder and clavicle injuries (continued)

Injury or condition	Mechanism of injury	Clinical presentation	Treatment
Shoulder dislocation	Violent rotation of the arm with the arm in abduction is the most common mechanism for shoulder dislocation. The shoulder can dislocate anteriorly, posteriorly and inferiorly, with the most common being anterior dislocation	• Obvious change (flattening) of shoulder contour • Severe pain • Holding arm to chest • X-ray confirms dislocation • Check for regimental badge sensation (axillary nerve) and for wrist drop (radial nerve)	• Analgesia • Prereduction X-ray to confirm diagnosis • Reduction of shoulder (various techniques) – only if trained to do so • Recheck neurovascular status • Postreduction X-ray • Immobilise collar and cuff or poly sling • Refer to fracture clinic
Acromioclavicular joint (ACJ) injury	Fall directly onto shoulder with arm adducted, direct blow or fall on an outstretched arm	• Superior shoulder pain • Reduced shoulder range of movement • ACJ swelling • Palpable step deformity to ACJ and/or elevated clavicle dependent on the grade of injury • X-ray may show widened ACJ or elevated clavicle at ACJ along the inferior border	• Analgesia • Broad arm sling • Refer to fracture clinic or physiotherapy as per local protocols
Soft tissue shoulder injury	Can be acute or chronic with causes ranging from muscular strain to impingement. Causes include heavy lifting, forced excessive range of movement and prolonged elevation of the arm	• Generalised shoulder pain • May have pinpoint tenderness dependent on the affected structure • Reduced range of movement • Painful arc indicating impingement	• Rest • Ice • Analgesia • Shoulder exercise advice • Referral to physiotherapy

Tibial/fibular injuries
Definition
Fractures to the tibia or fibula are commonly caused by direct blow; however other causes include falls from a height. Fibular fractures often accompany tibial fractures and can be caused by rotational forces.

History
• Identify the exact mechanism of injury.
• Identify function since injury.
• Identify other possible injuries.
• First-aid measures undertaken.
• Analgesia taken.

Tibial/fibular injuries (continued)
Examination
Look
- Inspect for swelling, bruising, wounds, deformity and colour of the skin.

Feel
- Palpate tibia and fibula and note the location of tenderness.
- Palpate the calf and note swelling and tenderness of the soft tissues.
- Examine the knee and ankle for injuries.
- Examine distal neurovascular status.

Move
- In proximal fibular fracture assess for ankle dorsiflexion weakness indicating injury to the peroneal nerve.

Investigations
- Tibial/fibular X-ray is the most useful imaging.

Management
Specific tibial/fibular injuries are discussed as follows:

Injury or condition	Mechanism of injury	Clinical presentation	Treatment
Tibial fractures	Direct blow to tibia, fall from a height or twisting forces	• Inability to weight bear • Swelling and bruising • Pinpoint bony tenderness • Visual deformity	• Analgesia • Long leg POP* • Referral to orthopaedics
Fibular fractures	Rarely isolated fracture and often accompanied by tibial fracture. Rotational forces are a common mechanism of injury	• May be able to partially weight bear • Swelling and bruising • Pinpoint bony tenderness	• Analgesia • Long leg POP* • Referral to orthopaedics
Maisonneuve fracture	A spiral fracture of the proximal fibula in addition to a fractured medial malleolus or ligamental injury. It is an unstable fracture associated with external rotation (This injury while uncommon reinforces the need to examine the proximal fibula in all ankle injuries)	• Unable to weight bear • Swelling and bruising to the medial malleolus • Swelling to the proximal fibula	• Analgesia • Long leg POP* • Referral to orthopaedics

*Placing patients that are non-weight bearing in below knee immobilisation is associated with increased risk of thromboembolism. Many centres now risk stratify for at-risk patients and provide appropriate prophylactic therapy.

Traumatic amputation
Definition
Traumatic amputation refers to accidental severing of a body part, either partially or complete. The extent of haemorrhage is dependent on the location of injury.

Aetiology
Common causes include RTCs, industrial and agricultural injury and gardening or DIY tools.

History
- Time of injury
- First-aid measures
- Past medical history
- Drug history
- Tetanus status

Investigations
- X-ray is indicated to assess extent of bone injury and the presence of radiopaque foreign bodies.

Management
- Manage as per ATLS guidelines as indicated.
- Analgesia (digital nerve block useful for digital amputation).
- Antibiotics as per local protocol.
- Consider the need for tetanus immunoglobulin.
- Refer to orthopaedic or plastic surgeons as per local protocols.

Remaining limb
- Control haemorrhage as necessary with pressure and elevation. In severe cases manage as per trauma guidelines.
- Elevate if possible.
- Loose tissue should be left in situ.
- Gentle cleaning with sterile saline and covered with moist sterile dressing.

Amputated part
- Wrap in sterile dressing and seal in plastic bag.
- Keep part cool by placing next to ice (tissue should not be in direct contact).

Upper limb injuries
Definition
Fractures to the humerus are often due to a fall and are common in older females due to osteoporosis. Biceps tendon rupture is secondary that occurs due to weakening secondary to repeated trauma or sudden and excessive loading.

History
- Identify the exact mechanism of injury.
- Identify the cause of fall (mechanical vs. collapse).
- Identify other possible injuries.
- Past medical and drug history.
- First-aid measures undertaken.
- Analgesia taken.

Examination
Look
- Inspect for swelling, bruising, wounds, deformity and colour of the skin.

Upper limb injuries (continued)
Feel
- Palpate and note the location of tenderness of the humerus bone.
- Palpate and note the location of tenderness of the upper arm soft tissues.
- Examine the shoulder and elbow.
- Check neurovascular status distally.

Move
- If fracture suspected do not move joint.
- Otherwise assess ROM at shoulder and elbow (active, passive and resisted).

Investigations
- Humerus X-ray is the most common method of imaging and is indicated when the mechanism of injury and clinical examination suggest bony injury. X-ray is not routinely indicated in suspected soft tissue injuries.

Management
Specific upper limb injuries are discussed as follows:

Injury or condition	Mechanism of injury	Clinical presentation	Treatment
Humeral head fractures	Low-energy fall in the elderly. High energy required in young patients. Females twice as likely to fracture head humeral head compared to men	• Swelling • Significant bruising • Deformity to the upper arm • Bony tenderness to proximal humerus • May have axillary nerve compromise	• Analgesia • Collar and cuff or broad arm sling • Refer to fracture clinic Nerve compromise or significant angulation should be discussed with orthopaedics
Humeral shaft fractures		• Swelling • Significant bruising • Deformity and tenderness to the humerus	• Analgesia • Collar and cuff or broad arm sling • Refer to fracture clinic
		May have radial nerve compromise	Nerve compromise or significant angulation should be discussed with orthopaedics
Rupture of the long head of the biceps tendon	Causes include repeated micro trauma leading to tendon weakness and rupture. Excessive load or rapid stress to the tendon can also cause rupture	• Sharp pain with tearing sensation • Pop-eye sign on contraction of the biceps • Often normal biceps strength • Swelling and bruising	• Rest, apply ice and reduce activity • Analgesia – paracetamol or NSAID • Referral to physiotherapy • Referral to orthopaedics for complete ruptures

(Continued)

Upper limb injuries (continued)

Injury or condition	Mechanism of injury	Clinical presentation	Treatment
Fracture of the mid-shaft of the radius and/or ulna	Direct blow to the forearm – common in assaults. Fall from height	• Often gross deformity • Swelling and bruising • Loss of forearm function Important: • High risk of compartment syndrome • Careful evaluation of distal neurovascular function required	• Analgesia • Discuss management with orthopaedic team as it often requires surgical intervention

Volar plate injuries
Definition
Volar plate injuries refer to a sprain to the ligaments of the volar plate with or without an avulsion fracture to the middle phalanx.

Aetiology
It is caused by forced hyperextension of the finger at the PIPJ.

History
• Mechanism of injury
• First-aid measures
• Analgesia

Investigations
• Finger X-ray is indicated to identify if avulsion fracture if present.

Management
• Rest.
• Apply ice.
• Elevate.
• Neighbour strapping.
• If no fracture present then refer to hand physiotherapy.
• If fracture present then refer to fracture clinic or hand surgeons as per local protocols.

Wrist injuries
Definition
Wrist fractures are common presentation to emergency and unscheduled care environments. They are often a result of the fall on the outstretched hand (FOOSH).

Age plays a significant part in the injury patterns as follows:

<10 years	Greenstick or buckle fractures
10–16 years	Salter–Harris fracture
17–40 years	Scaphoid fracture
40+ years	Colles' or Smith's fracture

Wrist injuries (continued)
History
- Identify the exact mechanism of injury.
- Identify function since injury.
- Identify other possible injuries.
- First-aid measures undertaken.
- Analgesia taken.

Examination
Look
- Inspect for swelling, bruising, wounds, deformity and colour of the skin.

Feel
- Palpate and note tenderness to the radial, ulnar and carpal bones.
- Palpate and note tenderness of the soft tissues.
- Examine the hand and elbow for injury.
- Check neurovascular status.

Move
- If fracture suspected do not move joint.
- Otherwise assess ROM – flexion, extension and ulnar and radial deviation.

Investigations
- Wrist X-ray is the most common method of imaging and is indicated when the mechanism of injury and clinical examination suggest bony injury. Obtain specific scaphoid views when scaphoid fracture is suspected.

Management
Specific wrist injuries are discussed as follows:

Injury or condition	Mechanism of injury	Clinical presentation	Treatment
Colles' fracture (fractured distal radius with dorsal displacement)	FOOSH – most common in patients over 40 years of age Often associated with ulnar styloid fracture	• Swelling and bruising to the wrist • Distal radial deformity – dorsal displacement (dinner fork) • Bony tenderness to the distal radius	• Analgesia • If displaced and angulated – reduction will be required • Below elbow back slab • Repeat X-ray • Broad arm sling • Referral to fracture clinic
Smith's fracture (fractured distal radius with ventral displacement)	Backward fall leading to FOOSH injury	• Swelling and bruising to the wrist • Distal radial deformity • Ventral displacement of distal fragment • Bony tenderness to the distal radius	• Analgesia • Discuss with orthopaedic team as it often requires surgical intervention • Below elbow back slab • Broad arm sling

(Continued)

Wrist injuries (continued)

Injury or condition	Mechanism of injury	Clinical presentation	Treatment
Wrist sprain	Often FOOSH injury but may also be due to carrying heavy objects or sudden extreme movement at wrist	• Pain and swelling to the wrist • Tenderness of the soft tissue • X-ray – no sign of bony injury • Stiff and general painful joint on movement	• Analgesia • Rest • Apply ice • Elevate • Wrist splint if required • Self-care management advice • Refer to physiotherapy if necessary or refer to GP if not improving
Wrist tenosynovitis (De Quervain refers to specific tenosynovitis to the thumb)	Swelling and inflammation of the tendon due to repetitive or prolonged strain	• Progressive pain and swelling • Discomfort exacerbated with wrist activity • Wrist stiffness • Palpable crepitus on tendon movement • Wrist weakness	• Wrist splint • Analgesia • Refer to GP if not improving in 2 weeks. Referral to physiotherapy may be required
Scaphoid fracture	FOOSH injury most common between 17 and 40 years of age	• Pain and swelling over anatomical snuffbox (ASB) • Tender ASB • Tender on telescoping thumb • Tender scaphoid tuberosity • Pain on flexion and ulnar deviation of the wrist • Scaphoid fractures often are not visible on initial X-ray • Diagnosis is therefore clinical with appropriate follow-up	• Analgesia • Broad arm sling Fracture confirmed on X-ray: • Below elbow back POP or splint (refer to local protocols) • Refer to fracture clinic No fracture seen on X-ray: • Below elbow back POP or splint (refer to local protocols) • Delayed appointment 10–14 days in fracture clinic for review
Carpal bone fracture	Often associated with high energy. FOOSH with wrist deviation or rotation	• Pain over carpals • Swelling • Reduced range of movement at the wrist Often difficult to see on X-ray – seek senior support	• Small avulsions or fractures can be placed in POP or split (refer to local protocols) • Refer to fracture clinic • Discuss with orthopaedic team if dislocation present

Neurology

Rapid Emergency and Unscheduled Care, First Edition. Oliver Phipps and Jason Lugg.
© 2016 John Wiley & Sons, Ltd. Published 2016 by John Wiley & Sons, Ltd.

Bell's palsy
Definition
Bell's palsy is defined as the idiopathic paralysis of the facial nerve (cranial nerve VII).

Epidemiology
It can affect up to 1 in 70 people. It affects men and women equally, although risk may be increased in diabetics and in pregnancy. Exact cause remains unknown and may be precipitated by viral, inflammatory, ischaemic or autoimmune causes.

History
- Sudden onset of weakness or complete paralysis of one side of the face
- Pain below the ear initially, which should subside. Early indication of Bell's palsy
- Difficulty swallowing
- Difficulty speaking
- Hyperacusis
- Impaired taste

Examination
- Unilateral facial weakness:
  - Inability to puff out cheeks, raise forehead and smile
- Inability to close the eye increases risk of infection, dry eye and the introduction of foreign bodies.
- Consider other causes of VII nerve palsy, for example, brainstem lesions, infection and systemic disease.

Investigations
- Diagnosis usually achieved through physical examination and history taking
- Imaging – indicated if there is doubt surrounding diagnosis or if treatment is prolonged:
  - CT
  - MRI
- Lumbar puncture – can be used to rule out other causes, for example, infectious processes

Management
- Discuss with senior clinician.
- Corticosteroids, ideally within 72 hours of symptoms.
- Antiviral drugs.
- Lubricating eye drops.
- Eye goggles or a patch may be beneficial.
- Psychological support.
- Refer to neurology.

House and Brackmann grading system (Sarhan et al., 2012)

Grade	Characteristics
I – Normal	Normal movement
II – Mild	Minor abnormalities including minimal synkinesis
III – Moderate	Symmetry at rest with mild disfigurement at movement; good eye closure

(Continued)

Bell's palsy (continued)

Grade	Characteristics
IV – Moderately severe	Symmetry at rest with gross disfigurement at movement; poor eye and forehead movement
V – Severe	Asymmetry at rest; minimal detectable function
VI – Total paralysis	No movement

From House, J.W. and Brackmann, D.E. (1985) Facial nerve grading system. Otolaryngol. Head Neck Surg, 93, 146–147.

Encephalitis
Definition
Encephalitis is an inflammation of the brain parenchyma, usually caused by a virus.

Epidemiology
It is most commonly caused by the herpes simplex virus (HSV) and is a rare disease which is more common in children, the elderly and those who are immunosuppressed. Approximately 2500 people in the United Kingdom develop encephalitis each year.

History
- Headache, which usually severe
- Nausea and vomiting
- Altered personality and confusion
- Lethargy
- Myalgia
- Fever
- Reduced consciousness
- Seizures

Examination
- Can be acutely unwell
- Meningitic signs (see 'meningitis')
- Reduced GCS
- Focal neurological signs
- Pyrexia
- Amnesia and hallucinations
- Bradycardic and hypertensive (signs of raised ICP)

Investigations
- Imaging:
  - CT head – urgent CT in those with focal neurology or seizures
  - MRI – may be more sensitive
- Lumbar puncture:
  - CSF pressure may be raised.
  - CSF PCR for HSV, varicella-zoster virus and enterovirus (covers ~90% of viral encephalitis cases).
  - CSF for lactate, cells, protein and glucose should also be examined.
- EEG
- Blood tests:
  - FBC, U&E, CRP and LFT – to exclude other potential sources
  - Blood cultures
- Consider non-infective causes of encephalopathy, for example, hepatic failure

Encephalitis (continued)
Management
- Refer to medical team.
- Manage the acutely unwell patient following an ABCDE approach:
  - Early referral to ITU for organ support
- IF HSV is suspected and acute illness present, then treat blindly with antiviral drugs.
- Antibiotic therapy if meningitis suspected.
- Corticosteroids.

Epilepsy
Definition
Epilepsy is a neurological condition in which recurrent abnormal electrical activity within the brain results in seizures. Seizures may be:
- Partial:
  - Simple partial seizure
  - Complex partial seizure
- Generalised:
  - Tonic–clonic seizure
  - Absent seizure
  - Tonic OR clonic seizure
  - Myoclonic seizure

Epidemiology
The prevalence of epilepsy is 5–10 per 1000 people. There is a slight increased incidence in the male population. Those with learning difficulties are at an increased risk. There is a 1% risk of having epilepsy at birth, compared to a 3% risk at the age of 75. Causes are generally idiopathic; however other pathologies such as cerebrovascular disease or head trauma can result in epilepsy.

History
- Witnessed seizure:
  - Witnesses may be crucial as generalised seizure caused disturbed consciousness.
- Blank spells
- Unexplained tongue biting
- Incontinence
- Hallucinations (may be visual, auditory or olfactory)
- Altered personality
- Prodrome or aura

Examination
- Ongoing seizure activity
- Generally normal neurology when not fitting
- Temperature – raised
- Tongue trauma
- Incontinence
- Head trauma

Investigations
- Imaging:
  - EEG – to support epilepsy diagnosis (note: a normal EEG is not a conclusive proof against a diagnosis of epilepsy)
  - CT/MRI head – to identify trauma/structural abnormalities/other pathologies

Epilepsy (continued)

- Blood tests:
  - FBC, U&E, LFT, CRP, calcium, magnesium and blood glucose – to exclude other causes of seizure
  - ABG – during or immediately post-seizure: raised lactate and low pO_2
- ECG – to exclude cardiogenic cause, for example, arrhythmia

Management

- Manage the acutely unwell patient following an ABCDE approach *(see status epilepticus)*.
- If first seizure occurs refer to 'first seizure clinic' as per local guidelines.
- Anti-epileptic drug therapy – aim for monotherapy, be guided by epilepsy specialists, monitor therapeutic levels and ensure concordance (refer to neurology).
- Advise against driving.
- Review regularly.
- Offer psychological support.

Giant cell arteritis

Definition

Giant cell arteritis is defined as an inflammatory disorder affecting the blood vessels.

Epidemiology

It typically affects branches of the carotid artery (temporal arteritis) and affects 1 in 10 000 people, more commonly in the elderly. It is rare in those under 55 years of age and tends to affect women more than men.

History

- Headache (often temporal)
- Altered vision
- Symptoms of polymyalgia:
  - Fever
  - Weight loss and anorexia
  - Proximal muscle stiffness and pain
  - Fatigue
- Jaw claudication

Examination

- Temporal artery and scalp tenderness
- Enlarged, pulseless temporal arteries
- Diplopia
- Amaurosis fugax (transient loss of vision in one eye)
- Pyrexia
- Carotid bruit

Investigations

- Blood tests:
  - FBC – low Hb and raised platelets
  - ESR – raised
  - CRP – raised
  - LFTs – raised alkaline phosphatase
- Imaging:
  - CT head – to exclude other pathologies
  - Chest X-ray – to exclude bronchial carcinoma
- Temporal artery biopsy

Giant cell arteritis (continued)
Management
- Start high-dose steroids immediately.
- Refer to neurology.
- Antiplatelet therapy.

Guillain–Barré syndrome
Definition
Guillain–Barré syndrome is an autoimmune disorder causing peripheral nerve inflammation and progressive ascending neuropathy, usually preceded by an infection.

Epidemiology
It is more common in males and affects 1–2 per 100 000 people per year. The majority of patients will have suffered a recent infection, usually gastric or respiratory, with the most common infection being campylobacter.

History
- Recent infection/vaccination/surgery.
- Progressive muscle weakness (usually starting in the lower limbs).
- Paraesthesia, usually starting in the hands and feet.
- Back or leg pain or cramps.
- Symptoms may progress rapidly.

Examination
- Reduced limb power (can be symmetrical or asymmetrical)
- Hypotonia
- Reduced peripheral sensation
- Abnormal cranial nerves
- Reduced or absent reflexes
- Diplopia
- Ataxia
- Autonomic dysfunction:
  - Tachycardia
  - Swinging blood pressure
  - Sweating
  - Fluctuating temperature
- Respiratory failure (in severe cases)

Investigations
- Bloods:
  - FBC, U&Es, CRP and LFTs – to exclude other causes of symptoms
- Lumbar puncture – CSF protein may be raised.
- Vital capacity – may be reduced.
- Nerve conduction studies.
- ECG – dysrhythmias can occur.
- CT head – to exclude another cause.

Management
- Urgent referral to hospital.
- Manage the acutely unwell patient following an ABCDE approach.
- Refer to neurology – may require plasma exchange or IV immunoglobulin.
- Refer to critical care – aim for early intubation if necessary.
- Closely monitor ECG and BP.
- Plasma exchange.
- DVT prophylaxis.
- Analgesia.

Meningitis
Definition
Meningitis is defined as an acute inflammation of the meninges (protective membranes which cover the brain and spinal cord). Four causes include bacteria, viruses, fungi and parasites.

Epidemiology
Meningitis occurs in all age groups, but the elderly and the young are more susceptible. Viral meningitis is the most common type, while bacterial meningitis is the most serious.

History
- Viral meningitis often mistaken for flu-like illnesses
- Headache (often sudden)
- Vomiting
- Photophobia
- Malaise
- Febrile

Signs of raised ICP:

- Drowsiness
- Seizures
- Coma
- Severe headache

Examination
- Kernig's sign +ve (pain and resistance on knee straightening during hip flexion)
- Brudzinski's sign +ve (flex head and neck and observe for hip flexion)
- Papilloedema
- Neck stiffness
- Petechial or purpuric rash
- Tachycardic, hypotensive and delayed capillary refill time (signs of sepsis)
- Bradycardic and hypertensive (signs of raised ICP)
- Decreased consciousness (more common with bacterial meningitis)

Investigations
- Urgent lumbar puncture (provided no signs of raised ICP):
  - May be normal in the early stages
- CT head (if signs of raised ICP, observe for signs of hydrocephalus or lesions)
- Bloods:
  - ABG (check for acidosis)
  - FBC, U&E, CRP and blood cultures
  - Clotting function (may indicate DIC)
  - Blood glucose (compare to CSF)
  - Polymerase chain reaction (PCR) test
- Chest X-ray (check for lung abscess)
- Skull X-ray (if history of recent head trauma)
- Urine, nasal swabs and stool cultures (for virology)

Management
- Manage the acutely unwell patient following an ABCDE approach.
- If signs of septicaemia are present, then treat before investigating (depending on local antibiotic guidelines).

Meningitis (continued)
- If outside of the hospital setting, treatment should always be commenced if meningitis is suspected (see local policy).
- Aim to identify organism and treat appropriately.
- Refer to intensive care if signs of shock are present (inotropic and ventilator support may be needed).
- Intravenous fluids.
- Viral meningitis:
  ○ Supportive treatment (antipyretics, analgesia, anti-emetics, hydration)

Migraine
Definition
Migraine is a chronic neurological condition which typically causes an aura followed by a severe headache.

Epidemiology
Women are affected more than men, with most migraine sufferers having experienced an attack before the age of 30. Migraines tend to peak in the fourth decade of life and often improve thereafter.

There are two main types:

1. Migraine with aura
2. Migraine without aura

There is often a family history of migraine.

History
- Known history of migraine
- Complaint of prodrome/aura:
  ○ Altered mood
  ○ Fatigue
  ○ Visual disturbance, for example, hemianopia
  ○ Paraesthesia
  ○ Dysphasia/dysarthria
  ○ Hemiplegia
- Headache – severe, interferes with daily activities, paroxysmal, usually unilateral, often pulsating
- Vomiting
- Photophobia
- Sensitivities to sound and smells
- Periodic abdominal pain and vomiting in children (abdominal migraine)

Examination
- A normal clinical examination may be found.

During attacks:

- Limb and facial paraesthesia
- Scalp tenderness
- Neck stiffness
- Limb ataxia
- Localised facial oedema

Investigations
- Only required if other pathologies are suspected

Migraine (continued)

> **Red flags**
> - Seizure
> - Altered consciousness
> - Papilloedema
> - Recent head trauma
> - Concurrent significant illness, for example, cancer
> - Sudden onset in those >50 or <10 years of age
> - Systemic symptoms
> - Any change in headache/aura which is not in keeping with the patients usual symptoms

- Imaging:
  - CT/MRI head if other pathologies are suspected

Management
- Anti-migraine drugs – triptans and ergotamine.
- Refer to neurology (if severe).
- Identify any triggers, for example, chocolate, cheese, stress, caffeine, oral contraceptives and alcohol.
- Analgesia and anti-emetics during attacks (may need to be PR).

Minor head injuries
Definition
Minor head injury is defined as a blunt or penetrating injury to the head or indirect trauma to the brain which does not cause significant illness but may cause transient altered neurological function (concussion).

Epidemiology
About 1.4 million people attend the Emergency Department in the United Kingdom each year with a head injury. Of these 50% are children and young people. The majority of these injuries are minor and leave no long-term disability. There is a slight increase in the incidence noticed in men. Falls, assaults and road traffic accidents account for the majority of head injuries.

History
- Recent trauma:
  - Risk of falls increases in the elderly
- Loss of consciousness
- Headache
- Dizziness
- Nausea
- Amnesia
- Confusion
- Poor balance
- Visual disturbances
- Recent alcohol consumption

Examination
- Visible injury
- GCS – may be transiently reduced but should return to baseline soon after injury
- Cranial nerves – should be normal (or return to normal soon after injury):
  - Diplopia or blurred vision may be present.

Minor head injuries (continued)
- Vital signs—should be normal
- Examine C-spine—to rule out traumatic injury

Investigations
- CT head if concerning neurological symptoms (refer to latest NICE guidelines).
- Vital signs.
- Blood glucose if indicated.
- Check GCS and repeat as necessary.

Management
- Analgesia.
- Patients with neurological symptoms will often need admission for observation.
- Reassure regarding normal symptoms and advise regarding red flags and the need to return.
- Explain and provide head injury information to patient and preferably another adult.
- CT head if indicated by NICE head injury guidance or on anticoagulants.
- Treat any soft tissue injuries.

Status epilepticus
Definition
Status epilepticus is defined as seizures lasting for longer than 30 minutes or repeated seizures which occur before the postictal phase ends. Status epilepticus is a medical emergency.

Epidemiology
Status epilepticus usually occurs in known epileptics, but non-epileptic seizures can result in status, for example, alcohol withdrawal, hypoglycaemia and drug withdrawal. Between ~10 and 60 presentations per 100 000 patients per year present in status. It is more common in the extremes of age.

History
- Seizure activity (see epilepsy) but unrelenting
- More common in known epileptics
- May be a history of alcoholism or substance misuse
- Potential head trauma

Examination
- Tonic–clonic seizures are easier to recognise.
- Non-convulsive status:
  - Subtle eye movements
  - Abnormal behaviour
  - Psychosis
  - Altered cognition
- Incontinence.
- Tongue biting.

Investigations
- Bloods:
  - Blood glucose—to rule out hypoglycaemic seizure
  - FBC, U&E, LFT, calcium and magnesium—to rule out other possible causes of seizure, for example, hyponatraemia
  - Anticonvulsant levels in known epileptics—may be subtherapeutic/toxic
  - ABG—usually a raised lactate and to exclude hypoxia as cause
- EEG
- CT head—to exclude brain lesion

Status epilepticus (continued)
Management
- Manage the acutely unwell patient following an ABCDE approach.
- Give high-flow oxygen.
- IV benzodiazepines:
  - Lorazepam 4 mg IV slowly or
  - Diazepam 10 mg IV slowly (can give PR if unable to gain IV access)
- Treat any reversible causes:
  - Hypoglycaemia – IV glucose
  - Alcohol excess – IV thiamine
- Contact ITU if seizures fail to terminate; may need anaesthesia and intubation.
- Phenytoin infusion.
- Seek expert advice.
- If seizures not terminating, consider pseudoseizures.

Stroke (cerebrovascular event)
Definition
Stroke (cerebrovascular event) is a neurological condition in which there is a disruption in the blood flow to the brain. There are two types:

1. Ischaemic – an occlusion of a vessel in the brain due to thrombosis or embolism
2. Haemorrhagic – the rupturing of a vessel either in the brain or on the surface

Transient ischaemic attacks (TIA) is the temporary occlusion of a cerebral vessel.

Epidemiology
Approximately 150 000 people suffer from a stroke in the United Kingdom every year. Around 70–80% of these are attributed to infarcts (ischaemic stroke), and around 15–20% are a result of haemorrhagic strokes. Men and women are equally affected. The risk of stroke increases significantly with age.

History
- Symptoms may be sudden or progressive.
- Slurred speech.
- Unilateral weakness.
- Confusion.
- Seizures.
- Incontinence.
- There may be a history of TIAs.
- Headaches (particularly in the case of subarachnoid haemorrhages).
- History of risk factors.

Risk factors
- Diabetes
- Atrial fibrillation
- Hypercholesterolaemia
- Hypertension
- Age
- Family history
- Smoking
- Peripheral vascular disease
- Clotting disorders
- Heart disease
- Contraceptive pill

Stroke (cerebrovascular event) (continued)
Examination
- Abnormal focal neurology/cranial nerves
- Hemiplegia
- Hemianopia
- Dysphasia
- Altered pupillary size and response
- Impaired cognition
- Ataxia
- Altered consciousness/locked-in syndrome
- Dysphagia
- Sensory loss
- Hypertension
- Think FAST (Face, Arms, Speech, Time)

Investigations
- CT head (urgently if acutely unwell or FAST positive)–to identify stroke or other causes of symptoms, for example, brain lesion
- Bloods:
  - Blood glucose–to identify other causes of abnormal neurology/consciousness
  - FBC–platelet abnormalities
  - ESR–raised in giant cell arteritis
- ECG–to identify potential arrhythmias that increase risk of emboli (e.g. AF)
- Echocardiogram–to rule out an atrial thrombus/valvular disease

Management
- Manage the acutely unwell patient following an ABCDE approach.
- Refer to hospital.
- Thrombolysis–if <4.5 hours since the onset of acute stroke and haemorrhagic stroke has been excluded.
- 300 mg aspirin PO/PR (if haemorrhage excluded).
- Nil by mouth.
- Correct blood sugar.
- Refer to ITU if airway is compromised.
- Discuss with neurosurgery with acute haemorrhages or if there are concerns about raised ICP.
- Refer to neurology.

Subarachnoid haemorrhage
Definition
Subarachnoid haemorrhage is the rupture of a blood vessel beneath the arachnoid membrane in the brain.

Epidemiology
Around 80% occur due to the rupture of an aneurysm within the circle of Willis (berry aneurysm), while 15% are secondary to arteriovenous malformations. Subarachnoid haemorrhages affect between 6 and 9 people per 100 000 per year, with women being at higher risk than men.

History
- Sudden severe headache, often occipital and thunderclap
- Neck stiffness
- History of trauma
- Altered consciousness/coma

Subarachnoid haemorrhage (continued)
- Nausea/vomiting
- 'Warning symptoms' or sentinel bleeds for weeks prior to the subarachnoid haemorrhage

Signs of raised ICP:

- Drowsiness
- Seizures
- Coma
- Severe headache

Examination
- Reduced GCS/coma.
- Bradycardic and hypertensive (signs of raised ICP).
- Abnormal neurological signs, for example, hemiparesis, unequal or unresponsive pupils and abnormal plantar responses.
- Intraocular haemorrhage.
- Neck stiffness (Kernig's +ve).
- Signs of external trauma may be present.
- Cardiac arrest occurs in 3% of patients.
- Pulmonary oedema (neurogenic) – rare.

Investigations
- CT head (ideally within 24 hours of onset) to identify subarachnoid or ventricular blood.
- Lumbar puncture – if CT head is negative. Perform >12 hours after onset of headache; if SAH is present then CSF should show xanthochromia.
- ECG – ST and rhythm changes can occur with SAH.
- Blood tests:
  ○ FBC, U&E, LFT and CRP – may indicate another cause for altered consciousness, for example, raised WCC, CRP and neutrophils in infection.
  ○ Clotting – observe for any coagulopathy.

Management
- Manage the acutely unwell patient following an ABCDE approach; intubation may be necessary.
- Refer to ITU for organ support.
- Refer to neurosurgery/interventional radiology:
  ○ Angiography – identify and coil aneurysm.
- Treat any seizures.
- Consider nimodipine to prevent vasospasm.
- Mannitol can be used to reduce intracranial pressure.
- Control hypertension.
- Bed rest.
- Monitor GCS and vital signs closely.

Subdural haemorrhage
Definition
Subdural haemorrhage is defined as an accumulation of blood beneath the dura mater which can be:
- Acute
- Subacute
- Chronic

Subdural haemorrhage (continued)
Epidemiology
It is most commonly associated with trauma. Up to one in three of those with serious head injuries may have a subdural haemorrhage. Those with arteriovenous malformations, aneurysms and clotting disorders are also at risk. Infants, the elderly and those with alcoholism are at an increased risk.

History
- History of trauma (note: the initial injury may have been minor and may have occurred weeks previously)
- Fluctuating consciousness
- Headache

Signs of raised ICP:

- Drowsiness
- Seizures
- Coma
- Severe headache

Examination
- Reduced GCS/coma.
- Bradycardic and hypertensive (signs of raised ICP).
- Abnormal neurological signs, for example, hemiparesis, unequal or unresponsive pupils and abnormal plantar responses.
- Papilloedema.
- Signs of external trauma may be present.

Investigations
- Imaging:
  - CT head – observe for subdural blood and midline shift.
  - MRI – may be more appropriate in chronic subdural haemorrhage due to better views.
- Blood tests:
  - FBC, U&E, LFT and CRP – may indicate another cause for altered consciousness, for example, raised WCC, CRP and neutrophils in infection.
  - Clotting – observe for any coagulopathy.

Management
- Manage the acutely unwell patient following an ABCDE approach.
- Seek senior clinician/critical care support.
- Refer to neurosurgery.
- Treat any seizures.
- Mannitol can be used to reduce intracranial pressure.
- Monitor GCS and vital signs closely.

Obstetrics and gynaecology

Rapid Emergency and Unscheduled Care, First Edition. Oliver Phipps and Jason Lugg.
© 2016 John Wiley & Sons, Ltd. Published 2016 by John Wiley & Sons, Ltd.

Eclampsia
Definition
Eclampsia is the end point of pre-eclampsia in susceptible women and is characterised by generalised convulsions (tonic/clonic).

Epidemiology
Eclampsia results in the death of 1000 babies and 10 women each year in the United Kingdom.

History
- Headache
- Photophobia
- Blurred vision or 'flashing lights'
- Abdominal discomfort
- Vomiting
- Disorientation
- Dizziness
- Jaundiced

Examination
- Decreased GCS
- Seizures
- Peripheral oedema
- Hypertensive
- Epigastric tenderness/abdominal pain
- Haemorrhage

Investigations
- Blood:
  - U&E
  - LFT
  - FBC
- Urine:
  - Urinalysis for protein

Management
- Airway management
- Oxygen
- IV access
- IV magnesium (avoid diazepam and phenytoin)
- Critical care

Ectopic pregnancy
Definition
Ectopic pregnancy is defined as a pregnancy sited outside the uterus, usually in a fallopian tube and is the most life-threatening of the early complications of pregnancy.

Epidemiology
The incidence of ectopic pregnancy is ~1% of all pregnancies. Ruptured ectopic pregnancies account for 13% of maternal deaths and are the leading cause of maternal death in the first trimester.

Ectopic pregnancy (continued)
History
- 5–8 weeks after the last menstrual period (LMP)
- Lower abdominal pain, often unilateral
- Vaginal bleeding
- Shoulder pain and hiccups are common
- Diarrhoea or pain on defecation
- Vomiting
- Feeling faint
- Low-grade pyrexia
- Signs and symptoms of shock

Note:
i. A history of previous ectopic pregnancy is a warning, as the condition often reoccurs
ii. Consider ectopic pregnancy in any women of childbearing age with abdominal pain

---

Examination
- Pale
- Lower abdominal pain
- Pain exacerbated on movement
- No or low-grade pyrexia
- Decreased GCS, tachypnoea, tachycardia and hypotension (if severe bleeding)

Investigations
- Bloods:
  - FBC – low Hb
  - U&Es – dehydrated
  - Clotting
  - HCG
- Urine:
  - HCG
- Imaging:
  - Transvaginal ultrasound (TVS)

If collapsed, perform abdominal FAST scan (to assess for intra-abdominal free fluid).

Management
If collapsed and/or haemodynamically compromised with suspected ectopic pregnancy:
- 999 ambulance to ED
- Urgent referral to obstetrics and gynaecology
- Large IV access × 2
- Fluid resuscitation
- Crossmatching
- Analgesia

Many patients present to emergency and unscheduled care environments with PV bleeding with or without abdominal pain that can be mild and unilateral and are haemodynamically stable. Suspicion arises of the possibility and need to exclude early ectopic pregnancy. In these circumstances it may be appropriate to:

- Refer to Early Pregnancy Assessment Clinic (EPAC) as per local protocols (discuss with gynaecology if unsure about suitability)
- Advise regarding analgesia and self-management
- Advise of red flags and the need to return

Hyperemesis gravidarum
Definition
Hyperemesis gravidarum (HG) is prolonged and severe nausea and vomiting, dehydration, ketosis and body weight loss in pregnancy.

Epidemiology
Around 7 in 10 women will experience nausea and vomiting in pregnancy until 14 weeks. It is thought that 1% of women are likely to develop HG.

> Other conditions in pregnancy can cause vomiting. Exclude genitourinary conditions such as urinary tract infection, pyelonephritis and ovarian torsion; endocrine conditions such as thyrotoxicosis, diabetic ketoacidosis and Addison's disease; gastrointestinal conditions such as gastritis, peptic ulcer, pancreatitis, bowel obstruction, hepatitis, cholelithiasis and appendicitis and neurological conditions such as vestibular disease and migraine. Also rule out other obstetric conditions.

History
- Nausea and vomiting.
- If vomiting begins after 9 weeks gestation, explore other causes.
- Fever and abdominal pain are not characteristic.

Examination
- Nothing found on clinical exam
- Dehydrated

Investigations
- Urine:
  ○ Urinalysis for ketones
- Imaging:
  ○ Consider pelvic ultrasound for predisposing molar pregnancy.

> Women with nausea and vomiting in pregnancy do not usually require laboratory evaluation unless symptoms are severe, prolonged (in terms of overall duration during pregnancy) or extended (in terms of frequency during each day).

Management
- Oral anti-emetic (off license – not licensed in pregnancy).
- Consider one dose of IM anti-emetic.
- Consider admission:
  ○ If symptoms are severe despite 24 hours of oral anti-emetic drug treatment (e.g. inability to tolerate liquids without vomiting)
  ○ There is evidence of dehydration, ketones in the urine or suspicion of medical complications

Miscarriage
Definition
Miscarriage is the death of a fetus or its spontaneous expulsion showing no signs of life, before 24 completed weeks of pregnancy.

Epidemiology
Miscarriage is unfortunately a common outcome of pregnancy, with 10–15% of confirmed pregnancies ending in miscarriage. This occurs most often at either 8 weeks or 12 weeks from the first day of the LMP.

Miscarriage (continued)
History
- Known pregnancy or late LMP.
- Known previous miscarriage.
- Abdominal pain may be present and cramping is most likely.
- Vaginal bleeding.
- Pregnancy tissue may have been expelled.

> Threatened miscarriage:
> Vaginal bleeding is associated with cramping abdominal pain, the cervix remains closed, and pregnancy may progress normally.
>
> Incomplete miscarriage:
> Vaginal bleeding may be heavy, the cervix is open, and abdominal pain is caused by uterine contractions, which have begun to expel the products of conception.
>
> Complete miscarriage:
> The products are completely expelled through an open cervix. Symptoms then settle.

Examination
- Pale.
- Possible tachycardia and hypotension.
- Generalised abdominal cramping.
- Pain can be variable.
- Vaginal bleeding.

Investigations
- Urine:
  - HCG to confirm pregnancy
- Imaging:
  - Consider pelvic ultrasound for predisposing molar pregnancy.

Management
- If there is small bleeding and patient is not compromised, allow home with referral to Early Pregnancy Assessment Unit (EPAU) the following day.
- If shocked:
  - Large IV access
  - Fluid resuscitate
  - Consider blood products
  - Discuss with O&G

Pre-eclampsia
Definition
Pre-eclampsia is pregnancy-induced hypertension with significant proteinuria.

Epidemiology
Pre-eclampsia can affect some pregnant women, usually during the second half of pregnancy (from around 20 weeks) or soon after their baby is delivered.

History
- Headache
- Photophobia
- Blurred vision or 'flashing lights'
- Abdominal discomfort
- Vomiting

Pre-eclampsia (continued)
- Disorientation
- Dizziness
- Jaundiced

Examination
- Hypertensive
- Epigastric tenderness

Investigations
- Blood:
  - U&E
  - LFT
  - FBC
- Urine:
  - Urinalysis for protein

Management

Mild (BP 140/90 to 149/99):
- Check renal function, FBC and LFTs.
- Refer to midwife and GP for management.

Moderate (BP 150/100 to 159/109):
- Bloods as aforementioned.
- Discuss with O&G.
- If CLINICALLY UNWELL consider antihypertensive therapy (oral labetalol).

Severe (BP > 159/109 or moderate pre-eclampsia with one of the following: headache; visual disturbance; severe subcostal pain; vomiting; papilloedema; clonus >3 beats; liver tenderness; haemolysis, elevated LFTs, and low platelet (HELLP) syndrome; platelets <100 × 10^9 and abnormal LFTs):

- Bloods as aforementioned.
- Urgent discussion with O&G.
- ICU referral.
- Urgent antihypertensive therapy.
- Treat as critical care patient.

Convulsion in pre-eclampsia:

- IV magnesium (do not use diazepam or phenytoin)

Vaginal bleeding (late pregnancy)
Definition
Third trimester vaginal bleeding (antepartum haemorrhage) is bleeding that occurs after 28 weeks of pregnancy.

Epidemiology
Vaginal bleeding in later pregnancy occurs in ~4% of pregnancies, with the two most common causes being:
- Placental abruption:
  The separation of a normally located placenta before delivery of the fetus. Bleeding occurs, and the blood is initially confined between the placenta and the uterine wall.
- Placenta praevia:
  Occurs when the placenta is implanted in the uterine segment, and subsequent separation will cause blood loss into the vagina. Bleeding will be heavy.

Vaginal bleeding (late pregnancy) (continued)
History
Placental abruption
- Abdominal pain of sudden onset
- With or without vaginal bleeding

Placenta praevia
- Vaginal bleeding

Examination
- Pale.
- Possible tachycardia and hypotension.
- Generalised abdominal cramping.
- Pain can be variable.
- Vaginal bleeding.

Investigations
- Bloods:
  - FBC = low Hb
  - Clotting
  - U&E
- Urine:
  - HCG to confirm pregnancy

Management
- Large IV access
- Fluid resuscitate if necessary
- Consider blood products
- Urgent referral to O&G

Ophthalmology

Rapid Emergency and Unscheduled Care, First Edition. Oliver Phipps and Jason Lugg.
© 2016 John Wiley & Sons, Ltd. Published 2016 by John Wiley & Sons, Ltd.

Acute angle-closure glaucoma
Definition
Acute angle-closure glaucoma is an increased intraocular pressure due to blockage of the flow of aqueous humour leading to damage of the optic nerve.

Aetiology
Blockages occur due to anatomical changes in the eye that commonly occur with ageing including thickening of the lens and narrowing of the iris. Medications which dilate the pupil may also precipitate acute glaucoma.

Epidemiology
It is more common in women than men and those with long-sighted vision. It commonly presents in the sixth and seventh decade of life and affects 1 in 1000 people a year.

History
- Pain – sudden onset (often occurs in the evening/night-time as the pupil dilates).
- Associated headaches and vomiting are common.
- History of visual disturbance (reduced visual acuity, blurred vision and halos).
- Previous history of glaucoma.
- History of new medications.

Examination
Perform a routine eye examination. Particular findings include red inflamed eye; tense globe to palpation; fixed, mid-dilated pupil and hazy cornea.

Investigations
- Test visual acuity.
- Measure intraocular eye pressures if available.

Management
- Urgent referral to ophthalmology for reduction of intraocular pressures with IV acetazolamide.
- Analgesia – patients may require intravenous analgesia and anti-emetics.
- If available, give pilocarpine eye drops to help constrict the pupil.
- Do not give any eye drops that will dilate the pupil further.
- Avoid darkened/dimmed rooms as this will cause the pupil to dilate.

Anterior uveitis
Definition
Anterior uveitis pertains to an inflammation of the anterior chamber of the eye. It may also be known as iritis or simply uveitis.

Aetiology
Inflammation commonly occurs due to an underlying autoimmune process which may or may not be identified. Infection and trauma can less frequently cause anterior uveitis. It often affects only one eye, but both eyes can be affected at the same time.

Epidemiology
It is commonly seen in patients with known autoimmune disorders such as ankylosing spondylitis, inflammatory bowel disease and reactive arthropathies.

History
- Pain – sudden onset
- Associated headaches

Anterior uveitis (continued)
- Light sensitivity and pain when focusing on objects
- Visual changes – blurred vision, change in visual acuity or new floaters

Examination
Perform a routine eye examination. Particular findings are as follows: the eye will be red and injected, commonly around the iris, and the pupil may be small or irregular.

Investigation
- Test visual acuity.
- Perform a slit lamp examination – this may reveal a hypopyon (pus in the anterior chamber) or visible inflammatory cells in the anterior chamber.

Management
- Analgesia – begin with oral analgesics.
- Mydriatic eye drops such as cyclopentolate will dilate the pupil and provide symptomatic relief.
- Refer urgently to ophthalmology for steroid therapy.

Blunt trauma
Definition
Blunt trauma is defined as a non-penetrative trauma to the eye, globe or socket.

Aetiology
Blunt trauma to the eye can result in a number of injuries to both the eye and surrounding bones, including subconjuctival haemorrhage, globe lacerations, lens dislocations, bony fractures including blow-out fractures, retrobulbar haemorrhage and retinal and vitreous bleeding or detachment.

Epidemiology
It is a common presentation to emergency departments typically in young males as a result of trauma from sporting injuries or assaults.

History
- Changes in vision are important as they may suggest retrobulbar haemorrhage, lens dislocation and retinal and vitreous haemorrhage or detachments.
- Double vision may indicate impingement of ocular muscles in bony fractures.
- A full history regarding possible head injury and any other injuries must be included.

Examination
- Perform a routine eye examination.
- Direct examination of the eye may reveal subconjunctival haemorrhages or abnormally shaped pupils.
- Pay particular attention to eye movements – these may be restricted if there is a bony injury to the orbit causing muscle impingement.
- Presence of proptosis suggests a retrobulbar haemorrhage.
- Examine the facial bones to exclude fractures.
- Check for paraesthesia of the face particularly in the infraorbital nerve distribution which may suggest a blow-out fracture.
- Perform a full examination of the head including neurological assessment to rule out associated intracranial injuries.
- Always consider possible cervical spine injuries.

Blunt trauma (continued)
Investigation
- Test visual acuity.
- Perform slit lamp examination with fluorescein to detect abrasions and visualise hyphaemas or globe lacerations.
- Fundoscopy may reveal a lens dislocation or vitreous/retinal haemorrhages or detachments.
- X-ray facial bones if tenderness is present.
- Perform a CT head scan if there are concerns about possible intracranial injury.

Management
- Refer patients with eye injuries secondary to blunt trauma to ophthalmology.
- Retrobulbar haemorrhage is an ophthalmological emergency and requires immediate referral to ophthalmology for sight-saving decompression.
- Manage patients with globe injury or hyphaema with head 45 degrees up.
- A joint referral to the maxillofacial surgeons may also be required if there is associated bony damage.

Chemical injury
Definition
Chemical injury includes injury to the eye resulting from chemical foreign body – may be acid or alkaline.

Aetiology
This is a very serious presentation which can lead to a severe chemical conjunctivitis and burns to the surface of the eye. Alkaline burns are likely to cause more damage than acid burns. These patients need to be assessed and managed urgently.

Epidemiology
Most cases will be as a result of work-related incidents although they are occasionally seen due to assaults, that is, acid attacks.

History
Important to elicit
- Substance
- Length of contact
- Initial first aid
- Contact lens wearers

Examination
- Examination should be brief as rapid irrigation may be sight saving.
- The eye is likely to be red, watery and inflamed.
- In extreme cases there may be opacification or even perforation of the cornea, which is a late and devastating sign.
- Do not delay irrigation to perform a detailed examination.

Investigation
- Test the pH of both eyes pre- and post-irrigation.
- Slit lamp examination with fluorescein.
- Visual acuity needs to be performed in time, but this should not delay irrigation.

Management
- The mainstay of emergency treatment is thorough and rapid irrigation of the eye with normal saline.
- Local anaesthetic eye drops may need to be administered first to aid this.

Chemical injury (continued)

- If the chemical agent is known, then a review of Toxbase is advisable for further advice.
- Refer immediately to ophthalmology.

Conjunctivitis

Definition

Conjunctivitis is an inflammation of the conjunctival surface of the eye causing watering and redness.

Aetiology

Common causes are viral, bacterial, chemical and allergic.

Epidemiology

Conjunctivitis is a very common presentation to the emergency department in all age ranges. Allergic conjunctivitis is likely to be seen more in the summer months.

History

- Is there an obvious trigger – infection, foreign body, or allergy?
- Is the discharge watery or purulent (this may help identify the underlying cause).
- Does the patient wear contact lenses?
- Patients often report a gritty or foreign body-type sensation in the eye due to irritation and inflammation.

Examination

- Perform a routine eye examination.
- The eye will be red and watery with or without purulent discharge.
- It is important to exclude a foreign body as an underlying cause particularly beneath the lids.

Investigation

- Test visual acuity.
- Perform a slit lamp examination with fluorescein to identify possible abrasions.
- Microbiology swabs are not routinely indicated.

Management

- Discharge the patient with chloramphenicol eye drops or ointment.
- Give advice on good eye hygiene.
- Conjunctivitis can be highly infectious; therefore infection control advice should be given.
- Advice patients not to drive if affecting visual acuity.

Corneal injury

Definition

Corneal injury is defined as a damage to the corneal surface commonly resulting in an abrasion.

Aetiology

It is often secondary to foreign bodies or direct trauma to the eye, that is, fingernail scratch

Epidemiology

It is the most common form of eye injury to present to emergency departments. It occurs in all ages and is most prevalent in contact lens wearers.

Corneal injury (continued)
History
- Red, painful and watery eye.
- Patients may have some light sensitivity.
- Patients often report a foreign body sensation.
- You must identify contact lens wearers.

Examination
- Perform a routine eye examination.
- Findings mainly include a red, inflamed and watery eye.

Investigation
- Test visual acuity
- Perform slit lamp examination with fluorescein staining which will identify abrasions and scratches.

Management
- Local anaesthetic drops will aid examination/investigation, but patients should not be discharged with them.
- Analgesia may be required.
- Discharge patients with chloramphenicol eye drops or ointment.
- Some patients may find an eye pad provides further symptomatic relief.
- Referral to ophthalmology is only required if there is ongoing symptoms after 36 hours.
- Advise patients not to drive until symptoms have settled.

Foreign bodies
Definition
Foreign body may become lodged on the cornea, conjunctiva or sub-tarsal area of the eye.

Aetiology
Foreign bodies easily enter the eye from the wind and air. They commonly collect in the lower fornix but may get stuck beneath the upper lid. Foreign bodies often cause irritation to the surface of the eye or lid resulting in conjunctivitis or a corneal abrasion. Some foreign bodies can enter the eye at high speed, that is, metal grinding resulting in globe penetration.

Epidemiology
It is a very common presentation to emergency departments and occurs in all age groups.

History
- Is the foreign body known/ is it metallic?
- Did it enter at speed?
- Could it have punctured the globe?
- Has the foreign body been removed?
- Are they wearing contact lenses?

Examination
- Perform a routine eye examination. The eye is likely to be red, watery and inflamed.
- Always invert the lids to check for hidden foreign bodies.
- Check for pupil irregularity which may suggest a penetrating injury.

Investigation
- Test visual acuity.
- Perform a slit lamp examination with fluorescein to identify abrasions, scratches or puncture wounds.

Foreign bodies (continued)

- In penetrating eye injuries a hyphaema or damage to the anterior chamber may be seen.
- X-rays of the globe may be indicated if a metallic foreign body has penetrated the globe.
- Consider fundoscopy to look for vitreous haemorrhage if a penetrating injury is suspected.

Management

- Use local anaesthetic eye drops to facilitate removal of foreign body with a cotton bud or 23G needle.
- Do not attempt to remove foreign bodies if there is a suspicion of penetration into the globe.
- Discharge on chloramphenicol eye drops or ointment.
- Referral to ophthalmology is not required unless there are ongoing symptoms after 36 hours or there is a residual rust ring.
- Urgent referral to ophthalmology and IV antibiotics with or without tetanus vaccination is indicated when penetrating eye injury is suspected.

Loss of vision

Definition

Loss of vision refers to sudden loss of vision in one or both eyes. This may be a complete loss or severe reduction in visual acuity, that is, finger counting/loss of light perception.

Aetiology

Most causes of loss of vision are a medical emergency and include central retinal artery or vein occlusion, TIA, optic neuritis and giant cell arteritis. Other common causes are vitreous haemorrhage or retinal detachments which can occur as a result of trauma or as a medical emergency.

Epidemiology

Most of these conditions are more common in the older patient who has other co-morbidities, particularly cardiovascular disease, cerebrovascular disease, diabetes or polymyalgia rheumatica. The exception to this rule is optic neuritis which is likely to present in young females.

History

- Enquire about history of trauma.
- Rapidity of onset of symptoms.
- Associated symptoms (headache, jaw pain, joint pains and other neurology).
- Identify risk factors and co-morbidities.

Examination

- Perform a routine eye examination.
- A relative afferent papillary defect may be present.
- Additional cardiovascular and neurological examinations may be indicated depending on the history.

Investigation

- Test visual acuity.
- Fundoscopy may reveal clues to the diagnosis.
- Bloods (FBC, UES, CRP, ESR, LFTs and clotting) may be indicated depending on the history.

Management

- Urgent referral to ophthalmology if ophthalmic diagnosis is likely.
- The aforementioned conditions all require rapid assessment, diagnosis and treatment by a senior doctor.

Subconjuctival haemorrhage
Definition
Subconjuctival haemorrhage refers to a well-defined collection of blood beneath the conjunctival surface.

Aetiology
This occurs due to increased venous pressure resulting in damage of small blood vessels. This can also occur as a result of trauma to the orbit or base of skull.

Epidemiology
It is seen more commonly in those with bleeding disorders or on blood-thinning medications. It is also more prevalent in patients with hypertension or diabetes.

History
- Often an incidental finding for the patient themselves!
- Some patients report a foreign body-like sensation in the eye on blinking.
- History of head or eye trauma may be important.

Examination
- Perform a routine eye examination.

Investigation
- Test visual acuity.
- A slit lamp examination may be indicated if there is a history of possible foreign body.

Management
Will resolve with no intervention in over 1–2 weeks

Superglue injuries
Definition
Superglue injuries pertain to superglue that has come into contact with the lids, lashes or surface of the eye.

Aetiology
When glue comes into contact with the eye, it causes a chemical conjunctivitis or keratitis. The glue will only bond to dry surfaces, that is, eyelashes.

Epidemiology
This is seen frequently in children and as a result of misidentification of bottles in adults. Unfortunately occasionally this also occurs iatrogenically when closing facial wounds with glue.

History
- What product has been used?
- How long has the glue been on?
- Do they wear contact lenses?

Examination
- Routine eye examination – the eye is likely to be glued closed by the lashes.
- If the eye has been opened, it will be red, watery and inflamed.

Investigation
- Slit lamp examination with fluorescein should occur once the eye is able to be opened to rule out abrasions caused by dry glue rubbing on the eye.

Superglue injuries (continued)
Management
- Soak with warm water to slowly dissolve the glue – this may take days to achieve.
- Trimming the eyelashes may aid eye opening.
- Refer to ophthalmology if evidence of abrasions is found late.

UV radiation injuries
Definition
UV radiation injuries include damage to the surface of the eye caused by ultraviolet radiation which are often referred to as arc welder's eye or superficial keratitis.

Aetiology
UVB radiation is absorbed by the cornea leading to damage which causes symptoms within a few hours. UVA radiation causes damage to the retina and macula, but this does not present acutely.

Epidemiology
It occurs in patients exposed to ultraviolet radiation – welders and sunbed users who have not used appropriate eye protection – or patients who have been in bright direct sunlight – something commonly seen in skiers.

History
Onset of painful watery eyes often occurs many hours after exposure.

Examination
- Perform a routine eye examination. This will show a red, inflamed and watery eye.

Investigation
- Test visual acuity.
- Slit lamp examination with fluorescein will show multiple punctuate lesions on the corneal surface of the eye.

Management
- Local anaesthetic eye drops will aid assessment, but patient should not be discharged with these.
- Give oral analgesia.
- Cyclopentolate eye drops can be given.
- Covering the eye helps improve symptoms.
- Patients must not drive while symptomatic.
- Ophthalmology follow-up is not required unless visual acuity has been affected.

Overdose and poisoning

Rapid Emergency and Unscheduled Care, First Edition. Oliver Phipps and Jason Lugg.
© 2016 John Wiley & Sons, Ltd. Published 2016 by John Wiley & Sons, Ltd.

Alcohol misuse and intoxication

Definition

Alcohol misuse and intoxication is a common problem particularly in emergency departments. Presentations attributed to alcohol may be physiological in nature, but often social and psychological issues are common. Patients who abuse alcohol often have various co-morbidities and reinforce the need for careful and accurate patient assessment.

Epidemiology

Exact epidemiological data varies, but some studies suggest that ~35% of all A&E attendances are alcohol related, increasing to around 70–80% at weekends.

History

- Routine alcohol questioning for all patients (e.g. Paddington Alcohol Test)
- Ascertain main reason for attendance (physiological, psychological or social)
- History of alcohol consumption (today vs. norm and when was last drink)
- Any trauma or physical symptoms
- Past medical and drug history
- Engagement with alcohol support services

Examination

- Patients with trauma or reduced level of consciousness have a high suspicion of discreet injuries – examine methodically.
- Vital signs – to identify abnormal physiology.
- GCS.

Investigations

There are no standard investigations required in alcohol misuse or intoxication. The need for bloods or imaging should be guided by the history and examination. Common investigations undertaken include:

- Blood glucose to exclude hypoglycaemia
- ECG – as indicated

Management

Acute intoxication

- If reduced level of consciousness, then manage with ABCDE approach and appropriate intervention.
- Manage in area where direct patient observation is possible.
- Assess for other injuries or pathologies – never assume presentation is primarily related to alcohol and manage accordingly.
- IV fluids can be helpful in speeding recovery.
- Discharge when patient safe with responsible adult.
- Consider referral to alcohol service if ongoing issue.

Alcohol withdrawal

- Manage seizure and tremor activity with benzodiazepines.
- Reverse hypoglycaemia as necessary.
- Exclude head injury.
- Manage withdrawal with benzodiazepines, parenteral thiamine and multivitamins.
- Refer to local protocols regarding ongoing management of alcohol withdraws.

Carbon monoxide poisoning
Definition
Carbon monoxide is a colourless, odourless, tasteless gas produced by incomplete combustion of organic material. Acute exposure causes tissue hypoxia due to its higher affinity for haemoglobin than oxygen. This leads to impaired cell function and can cause tissue damage.

Epidemiology
It is estimated that around 50 deaths occur annually in the United Kingdom due to carbon monoxide poisoning with a further 200 incidences requiring hospital admission.

History
- Headache
- Lethargy
- Dizziness
- Nausea, vomiting and diarrhoea

More severe symptoms include:

- Vertigo and ataxia
- Impaired mental state
- Chest pain
- Breathlessness and tachycardia
- Seizures

Examination
- CVS, respiratory and CNS examination as minimum

Investigations
- Vital signs (temp, RR, HR, BP and SpO_2).
- Blood glucose to exclude hypoglycaemia.
- ECG if chest pain or tachycardic.
- Arterial or venous blood gas for COHb levels >10% definitively indicates poisoning (1–2% normal and 5% normal in smokers).

Management
- Remove from source.
- 999 ambulance to ED if prehospital.
- High flow oxygen.
- Treat symptomatically and monitor until asymptomatic and COHb levels are within the normal range.
- Advise not to return to property if identified cause until air levels are checked and deemed safe.

Note: the half-life of carboxyhaemoglobin is 320 minutes – with high flow oxygen this is reduced to 80 minutes.

Drug misuse
Definition
Drug misuse is a common problem particularly in emergency departments. Presentations can vary and include physiological, psychiatric and social incidents. There is a significant range of recreational drugs, with changing street names. Toxbase provides a useful reference source on typical presentation and management.

Drug misuse (continued)
Epidemiology
Research undertaken in 2010–2011 revealed that the prevalence for ever taking illicit drugs in England and Wales was 36%, with 8% having taken one or more illicit drugs in the last year and 3% having taken a class A drug in the last year.

History
- Routine recreational drug questioning for all patients is good practice and should be asked as part of history taking.
- Ascertain main reason for attendance (physiological, psychological or social).
- History of drug use (drugs used, normal pattern, route, etc.).
- Past medical and drug history.
- Engagement with drug support services.

Examination
- ABCDE approach.
- Examination will be directed by reason for presenting. It is important to assess carefully and refrain from a judgemental approach. Patients with trauma or reduced level of consciousness have a high suspicion of discreet injuries – examine methodically.

Investigations
- Vital signs (temp, RR, HR, BP and SpO_2)
- GCS
- Blood glucose
- ECG
- Bloods – as indicated

Management
- If acutely unwell manage with ABCDE approach with interventions as required.
- Refer to Toxbase for specific adverse effects, investigations and management.

Specific considerations of common drugs include:

Drug	Effects	Presentation	Treatment
Heroin (opioid)	CNS depression: drowsiness, coma, respiratory depression and respiratory arrest	Pinpoint pupils and reduced respiratory rate, hypotension	ABCDE support and naloxone IV, IM or intra-nasal
Cocaine	Induces euphoria and excitement by blocking the reuptake of dopamine	Agitated, sweating, dilated pupils, hypertension and chest pain	Treat symptomatically, ECG, aspirin and IV diazepam in chest pain (avoid β-blockers)
Ecstasy (MDMA)	Psychoactive drug with hallucinogenic effects	Sweating, dilated pupils, tachycardia, hypertension and in severe cases hyperthermia	Treat symptomatically and with IV diazepam and IV fluids as required

Paracetamol overdose
Definition
Overdose is a term used to describe the use of a quantity of drug in excess of its intended or prescribed dose. Paracetamol overdose is common due to its widespread availability. Overdose may be accidental or deliberate, with accidental overdose occurring due to errors in drug administration or polypharmacy.

Paracetamol overdose (continued)
Epidemiology
Paracetamol represents one of the most frequently used drugs for intentional overdose. In the United Kingdom it accounts for around 48% of poisoning admissions with a mortality of between 100 and 200 patients per year.

History
- Ascertain why the paracetamol was taken – was it accidental or deliberate?
- What exactly was taken? Look at containers or packets if possible.
- How much was taken?
- Was any other medicines, substances or alcohol taken?
- When was the exact time the paracetamol was taken?
- Was it taken over less than or greater than 1 hour?
- Emotional and mental state now? Any continuing suicidal intent?
- Nausea and vomiting (usually settles in around 24 hours).
- Abdominal pain.
- Past medical history.
- Drug history.
- Allergies.

Examination
- Cardiovascular, respiratory, abdominal and neurological examination (in early stages of poisoning examination will be normal).
- Note specifically liver tenderness or jaundice (indicates hepatic necrosis).
- Mental health matrix assessment if deliberate.

Investigations
- Vital signs (temp, RR, HR, BP and SpO_2).
- Blood glucose.
- Weight.
- Bloods (FBC, U&Es, LFTs, INR, paracetamol levels) – the timing is dependent on the time, whether staggered and ingested dose mg/kg (please refer to current guidelines). If ingestions were <4 hours ago, then delay bloods until 4 hours post-ingestion time.
- Venous blood gas.

Management
- Refer to ED if prehospital.
- Bloods as per above.
- Immediately start N-acetylcysteine (NAC) if:
  - Single ingestion >15 hours ago.
  - Staggered ingestion (taken over >1 hour) – NAC should be started within 1 hour of ED arrival.
  - Significant ingestion >4 hours ago (>75 mg/kg).
  - *Otherwise wait for 4 hours post-ingestion blood results – refer to latest clinical guidelines on Toxbase.*
- Refer to mental health services if deliberate.
- IV anti-emetics.
- Refer to ED observation unit or medical team as per local protocol

Poisoning
Definition
Poisoning is the administration of a substance, taken internally or externally, that causes injury or danger to life. Poisons vary from drugs, plant products, household products and industrial chemicals. Poisoning may be accidental or intentional with accidental poisoning occurring due to domestic accidents, workplace exposure or environmental incidents.

Poisoning (continued)
History
- Determine the exact circumstances of the poisoning information from friends and family.
- Why was the substance taken – accidental or deliberate?
- Past medical history (identify any factors that will affect the excretion or metabolism of the poison – renal or hepatic impairment).
- What was taken? Look at containers where possible.
- Route of administration – ingested, inhaled or injected.
- If deliberate – assess emotional and mental state and continued suicidal intent.

Examination
- System examination (CVS, respiratory, abdominal, CNS and skin) – guided specifically by likely poison effect

Investigations
- Vital signs (temp, RR, HR, BP and SpO_2).
- Other investigations need to be guided by the likely effect of the poison.

Management
- Remove source.
- 999 ambulance to ED if prehospital.
- Refer to Toxbase to ascertain specific poison mechanism of action, investigations required and treatment.

Respiratory

Rapid Emergency and Unscheduled Care, First Edition. Oliver Phipps and Jason Lugg.
© 2016 John Wiley & Sons, Ltd. Published 2016 by John Wiley & Sons, Ltd.

Asthma
Definition
A chronic inflammatory condition of the airways, characterised by variable reversible airway obstruction, hyper-responsiveness and bronchial inflammation.

Aetiology
Precipitating factors: weather, viral infection, drugs, exercise and emotions
Genetic factors: positive family history
Environmental factors: house dust mite, pollen, pets, smoking, viral respiratory infections and fungus

Epidemiology
Asthma prevalence is increasing, with ~10% of children and 5% adults, with equal gender distribution. Acute asthma is very common and is still responsible for 1000–2000 annual deaths in the United Kingdom.

History
- Wheeze
- Breathlessness
- Cough
- Worse at night and early morning
- Exercise difficulty
- Previous asthma attack history, hospital admissions and intensive care admissions

Examination
Raised RR, use of accessory muscles, tachycardia, prolonged expiratory phase, wheeze and hyperinflated chest

Severe
- Incomplete sentences
- PEFR <50% of best
- Tachycardia
- Tachypnoea

Life threatening

- Silent chest
- PEFR <33% of best
- Poor respiratory effort
- Cyanosis
- HR <60 bpm or >120 bpm
- Confusion
- SpO_2 <92%
- pO_2 <8 kPa
- Tiredness/exhaustion
- Systolic BP <100 mmHg

Near fatal
- CO_2 retention

Investigations
Acute
- Peak flow
- ABG (hypoxia and hypercapnia)
- CXR (to exclude causes)
- Blood: FBC, CRP (for infection markers) and U&Es
- Cultures if pyrexia
- Atypicals

Asthma (continued)
Chronic
- Peak flow
- Pulmonary function tests
- Blood: eosinophilia and aspergillus
- Skin prick testing – allergen identification

Management
Acute
- Sit up.
- Salbutamol nebuliser (back to back via O_2).
- Ipratropium.
- IV hydrocortisone.
- Consider IV magnesium.
- Senior help.

Chronic
- BTS step approach:
  - Lifestyle coaching and allergen advice.
  - Increase inhaler dose.
  - Add corticosteroid inhaler.
  - Consider oral prednisolone.
  - Consider long-acting beta-agonist.
  - Consider antibiotics.

Chest sepsis (including pneumonia)
Definition
An acute infection of the lower respiratory tract associated with fever and other chest signs and symptoms.

Epidemiology
A common presentation with 1–3/1000 affected and a mortality rate of 10%. Pneumonia can be community acquired, hospital acquired, following aspiration and when immunocompromised.

History
- Community acquired:
  - Can be associated with underlying disease
  - Previous respiratory illness, infection, influenza or coryza
- Hospital acquired:
  - >48 hours admission
  - Usually associated with long length of stay
- Aspiration:
  - Poor swallow
  - Stroke, myasthenia, bulbar palsies, decreased level of consciousness and post-anaesthetic
- Immunocompromised

Examination
- Fever, rigors and malaise
- Dyspnoea, cough and productive sputum
- Possible pleuritic pain
- Tachypnoea, tachycardia and possible hypotension

Chest sepsis (including pneumonia) (continued)
- Chest:
  - Dull percussion
  - Crackles
  - Increased tactile vocal fremitus
  - Pleural rub

Investigations
- Bloods:
  - FBC (increased infection markers)
  - CRP (raised)
  - U&Es (urea can be raised)
  - Liver function
- Arterial blood gas (hypoxia, hypercapnia)
- Sputum culture
- Chest X-ray:
  - Consolidation
  - Pleural effusion
- Use CURB-65 tool to mark severity:
  - Confusion
  - Urea >7 mmol/l
  - Respiratory rate >30 bpm
  - Blood pressure (SBP) <90 mmHg
  - Age ≥65 years
- <2 consider treating at home
- 2 hospital admission
- ≥3 severe

Management
- If well:
  - Oral Abx.
  - Encourage oral fluids.
- If unwell:
  - Resuscitation (direct to emergency department).
  - ABCDE approach.
  - Oxygen (set SpO_2 target).
  - IV access.
  - IV fluid.
  - IV antibiotics.
  - Analgesia.
  - Consider ICU.

Chest wall injury
Definition
Chest wall injuries are extremely common following blunt trauma. They can vary in severity from minor bruising or an isolated rib fracture to more severe injuries, leading to respiratory compromise.

Epidemiology
Chest wall injuries are commonly seen in the urgent care setting.

History
- When did the injury occur?
- Consider mechanism of injury.

Chest wall injury (continued)

- Any risk of penetrative trauma?
- Any shortness of breath?
- Pain on inspiration or chest movement?
- Any haemoptysis?
- Smoking history.

Examination

- ABCDE approach – perfusion and respiratory rate.
- Is the patient pale – bleeding?
- Is trachea central and is there any chest deformity?
- Equal chest movement (rise/fall).
- Bruising, marks and flail segment?
- Respiratory exam:
  - Respiratory distress
  - Equal breath sounds
  - Hyper-resonance on percussion
- Tenderness on palpation
- Surgical emphysema

Investigations

- Vital signs – RR, HR, BP (both arms) and SpO_2
- 12-lead ECG
- CXR (consider need depending upon clinical signs)
  - To identify and exclude a pneumothorax or haemothorax
  - If sternal fracture request a lateral sternal X-ray
- Bloods and ABG in serious chest trauma

TOP TIP:
- 50% of isolated rib fractures are not visible on a CXR.
- Treat a tension pneumothorax if suspected first, then CXR.

Management

- Severe:
  - Prepare to resuscitate.
  - Oxygen and IV access.
  - Analgesia.
  - Urgent senior review/critical care support/thoracic surgeons.
    - Think: chest drain, intubation and ventilation.
- Minor:
  - Analgesia.
  - Deep breathing exercises (to prevent a developing chest infection).
  - Discharge (vital signs should be normal).
  - Seek medical advice if developing breathlessness, feeling unwell or increased pain.

Chronic obstructive pulmonary disease (COPD)
Definition

A chronic lung disorder, characterised by airflow obstruction and encompassing chronic bronchitis and emphysema.

Chronic bronchitis: a chronic cough and sputum production for at least 3 months per year, over two consecutive years.

Emphysema: pathological diagnosis of permanent destructive enlargement of air spaces distal to the terminal bronchioles.

Chronic obstructive pulmonary disease (COPD) (continued)
Aetiology
Caused by environmental toxins (cigarette smoking), and alpha one – antitrypsin deficiency, a rare condition which should be considered in the young and non-smokers.

Epidemiology
A very common condition (up to 8% prevalence). Presents in middle age or later and more common in males at present. Approximately 30 000 deaths each year.

History
- Chronic cough and sputum production
- Breathlessness
- Wheeze
- Poor exercise tolerance

Examination
Inspection
- Barrel-shaped chest
- Hyperinflated chest
- Decreased cricosternal distance
- Cyanosis
- Respiratory distress
- Accessory muscle use

Percussion
- Hyper-resonant chest
- Loss of liver and cardiac dullness

Auscultation
- Quiet breath sounds
- Wheeze
- Prolonged expiratory phase
- Reduced air entry
- Rhonchi
- Crepitations

Other
- CO_2 flap (hand tremor)
- Bounding pulse
- Right heart failure in later stages (raised JVP/ankle oedema)

Investigations
- CXR (could show hyperinflation)
- Pulmonary function tests (looking for an obstructive picture and low $FEV_1 : FVC$ ratio)
- Bloods FBC and CRP (infection markers in an exacerbation)
- ABG (hypoxia/hypercapnia)
- ECG and echo (for cor pulmonale)
- Sputum and cultures (infection sensitivities)

Management
Acute exacerbation (*refer to local and national guidelines*)
- IV access
- Oral/IV antibiotics
- Oral/ IV steroids

Chronic obstructive pulmonary disease (COPD) (continued)

- Controlled oxygen
- Nebulised bronchodilators
- IV aminophylline
- Non-invasive ventilation in type 2 respiratory failure
- Ceiling of care
- Referral to ICU if appropriate

Chronic management (*refer to local and national guidelines*)

- Bronchodilators
- Inhaled steroids
- Oral steroids
- Oxygen
- Mucolytics
- Vaccinations
- Consider palliative care referral for anxiety management

Croup (acute laryngotracheobronchitis)
Definition
A barking cough, stridor and low-grade pyrexia, often associated with an upper respiratory illness. This is an inflammatory process extending to the vocal chords and epiglottis.

Epidemiology
Often seen in children between 6 months and 6 years. Children <3 years are most severely affected.

History
- Viral illness over few days
- Pyrexia
- Barking cough
- Generally unwell

Do not distress the child. Keep child on parents lap if distressed, and avoid invasive investigations/treatment unless absolutely necessary.

Examination
- Generally unwell
- Mild pyrexia
- Barking cough
- Coryzal symptoms
- Occasional stridor
- Inflamed throat
- In severe cases:
  - Stridor
  - Cyanosis
  - Intercostal recession
  - Respiratory distress

Caution: This could be epiglottitis! Call for senior help and avoid irritating the airway.

Croup (acute laryngotracheobronchitis) (continued)
Investigations
- Avoid investigation, as this will distress the child, if possible.

Management
Mild
- Oral dexamethasone.
- If no evidence of respiratory distress and child interacting normally, consider discharge.

Moderate/severe
- ABCDE approach.
- Consider oxygen.
- Consider nebulised steroids and adrenaline.
- Senior help (paediatrician and anaesthetist)
  - Admit if signs of respiratory distress, cyanosis, severe stridor or fatigue.
  - Intensive care support and early intubation.

> Consider epiglottitis!

Cystic fibrosis
Definition
An autosomal recessive inherited multisystem disease characterised by multiple recurrent respiratory tract infections, malabsorption, pancreatic insufficiency and male infertility.

Aetiology
Caused by a defective CFTR gene on chromosome 7q.

Epidemiology
Most common autosomal inherited condition in white people; 1/2500 live births in the United Kingdom, with 1/25 being carriers.

History
- Recurrent chest infections
- Chronic cough and wheeze
- Sputum
- Chronic sinusitis
- Arthritis
- Steatorrhoea
- Weight loss

Examination
Chest: chest wall deformity with coarse crepitations and wheeze
Abdomen: hepatomegaly and signs of diabetes
Other: clubbing
Signs of: anaemia, vitamin deficiency and delayed puberty

Investigations
- CXR (normal in mild disease, developing bronchial markings and ring shadowing; consolidation with or without bronchiectasis in advanced cases).
- Pulmonary function testing – predetermine long-term prognosis.
- Pancreatic Assessment – faecal elastase and fat content, HbA1c and GTT.
- Genetic analysis for CFTR mutations.

Cystic fibrosis (continued)
Management
Specialist management is required from the MDT.

Respiratory care
- Physiotherapy (postural drainage)
- Bronchodilators (if effective)
- Antibiotic prophylaxis
- Flu vaccination

Gastroenterology
- Dietician support
- High-calorie supplements
- Oral pancreatic enzyme replacement
- Vitamin supplements

Endocrine
- Diabetes management and insulin replacement if necessary

Flail chest
Definition
Two or more adjacent ribs are broken in two places resulting in a flail segment which moves paradoxically on inspiration (in on inspiration and out on expiration).

History
- Chest trauma
- Compression of chest
- Blunt trauma
- Associated with road traffic collisions (usually unrestrained) and falls

Examination
- Breathlessness
- Chest pain
- Tender chest on palpation
- Look at chest in detail from patient's feet:
  - Paradoxical breathing
  - Dynamics of breathing
  - Poor 'rise and fall'

Investigations
- Do not delay treatment.
- CXR.
- ECG.
- ABG (hypoxia/hypercapnia – tiring).

Management
- Sit up.
- 15 l O_2 via non-rebreather mask.
- Urgent transfer to emergency department – consider major trauma.
- Analgesia.
- Observe for tension pneumothorax or tiring.

Haemothorax
Definition
Blood in the pleural space, with no means of escape.

Epidemiology
Associated with blunt and penetrating trauma.

History
- Chest trauma:
  - Blunt trauma (fall, road traffic collision, assault)
  - Penetrating trauma (stabbing)
- Post-operative

Examination
- Can be asymptomatic
- Breathlessness
- Chest pain
- Decreased air entry on the affected side
- Dull percussion over the affected side
- Tachycardia, hypotension and signs of shock
- Low jugular venous pressure

Investigations
- If clinically stable:
  - CXR

Management
- Sit up.
- 15 l O_2 via non-rebreather mask.
- IV access.
- IV fluid resuscitation (to maintain radial pulse).
- Urgent transfer to emergency department – consider major trauma.

Lung cancer
Definition
Primary malignancy of the lung.

Epidemiology
Most common fatal malignancy in the West; 35 000 UK deaths per year; three times more common in men.

History
- Can be asymptomatic
- Primary:
  - Cough, haemoptysis, chest pain and reoccurring chest infection
- Metastatic:
  - Weight loss
  - Fatigue
  - Bone pain
  - Seizures

Examination
- No signs or symptoms
- Fixed monophonic wheeze

Lung cancer (continued)
- Signs of pleural effusion or lobar collapse
- Lymphadenopathy or hepatomegaly

Investigations
- CXR
- Sputum

Management
- Multidisciplinary input
- Respiratory physician referral:
  - Bronchoscopy
  - Staging CT
  - CT biopsy
  - Lymph node biopsy

Open chest wound: Medical emergency
Definition
An open pneumothorax, which can be described as a 'sucking chest wound'.

Epidemiology
Commonly follow stab and gunshot wounds, although present following road traffic collisions and industrial accidents.

History
- Chest trauma
- Polytrauma

Examination
- Visible large chest wound:
  - If greater than two thirds the diameter of the patient's trachea air will pass through the wound preferentially.
- Respiratory distress
- Tachycardia, hypotension and shock

Investigations
- Do not delay treatment.

Management
- Sit up.
- 15 l O_2 via non-rebreather mask.
- Asherman® chest seal or a dressing with three edges sealed (fourth edge open).
- Do not seal all four edges, as tension pneumothorax will occur.
- Be prepared to needle-decompress if tension pneumothorax develops.
- Emergency transfer to emergency department – consider major trauma.

Pulmonary embolism
Definition
An occlusion of the pulmonary vessels, most likely by a thrombus that has travelled through the vascular system from another site.

Epidemiology
Relatively common, 10–20% of those with a confirmed proximal DVT.

Pulmonary embolism (continued)
History
- Breathlessness and/or tachypnoea
- Pleuritic chest pain (not always)
- Haemoptysis (not always)

Risk factors:
- Recent surgery
- Recent thrombolic event
- Disseminated malignancy
- Immobility
- Pregnancy
- Medication – OCP

Examination
Raised RR, raised JVP, tachycardia, hypotension and pleural rub

Investigations
If low probability consider D-dimer blood test (sensitive, but poor specificity).

Wells score for PE	
Previous PE or DVT	1.5
Heart rate >100 bpm	1.5
Surgery or immobilisation within 30 days	1.5
Haemoptysis	1
Active cancer (within 6 months)	1
Clinical signs of DVT	3
Alterative diagnosis less likely than PE	3
PE low risk = 4 and below	
PE high risk = 4.5 and above	

D-dimer can be positive with cancer, infection, inflammation, arthritis, necrosis, aortic dissection, pregnancy, trauma and surgery.

If high probability refer for imaging. CT pulmonary angiogram is the first-line investigation of choice (poor sensitivity for small emboli, but very sensitive for medium and large emboli).

Additional investigations
- FBC and U&Es for baseline.
- ABG may show a low pO_2 and a low pCO_2.
- CXR may be normal or could show dilated pulmonary artery, linear atelectasis or oligaemia.
- ECG may be normal or tachycardia, RBBB, inverted T waves and S1Q3T3 phenomenon.

Management
Chronic treatment
- Warfarin for 6 months or for life if second episode

Acute treatment
- Sit up and give 15 l O_2.
- LMWH (treatment dose).
- Fluid resuscitate if hypotensive.
- Analgesia.

If life threatening
- CTPA or echo followed by thrombolysis

Pneumothorax (simple)
Definition
Air in the 'potential', pleural space.

Pneumothorax (simple) (continued)
Epidemiology
Common presentation in sport players, especially young men.

History
Primary risk factors: tall, thin and male
Secondary risk factors: COPD, asthma, infection, trauma, recent medical procedures (central line/chest aspiration), mechanical ventilation and non-invasive ventilation
Breathlessness with or without chest pain

Examination
Raised RR, hyper-resonance, reduced air entry and breath sounds on affected side, may have tracheal deviation and rib fractures

Investigations
- CXR
- ABG if hypoxic
- Pleural ultrasound

Management
- Sit up.
- Chest aspiration or chest drain (see BTS guidelines)

Tension pneumothorax: Medical emergency
Definition
Air in the pleural space, increasing with each breath with no means of escape.

History
Chest trauma, COPD, asthma, recent medical procedures (central line/chest aspiration), mechanical ventilation and non-invasive ventilation
Breathlessness, chest pain and hypovolaemic collapse

Examination
Respiratory distress, tachycardia, hypotension, distended neck veins and deviated trachea (away from pneumothorax)

Investigations
- Do not delay treatment.
- CXR post-needle decompression.

Management
- Sit up.
- 15 l O_2 via non-rebreather mask.
- Needle decompression:
  - 14–16G cannula inserted into the *second intercostal interspace in the mid-clavicular line* on the side of the suspected pneumothorax.
  - Following this a chest drain will be required.

Skin

Rapid Emergency and Unscheduled Care, First Edition. Oliver Phipps and Jason Lugg.
© 2016 John Wiley & Sons, Ltd. Published 2016 by John Wiley & Sons, Ltd.

Abscesses
Definition
A mass of necrotic tissue with dead and viable neutrophils suspended in pus, which is surrounded by inflammatory exudate.

Epidemiology
Common in all ages.

History
- Pain
- Redness, swelling and heat
- Impaired function
- Fever
- Flu-like symptoms

Examination
- Acute inflammation can be seen at the site of the abscess.
- If internal (within an organ):
  - Swinging pyrexia
  - Presents generally unwell

Investigations
- Bloods – FBC (raised neutrophils) and CRP (raised)
- Imaging – ultrasound or CT
- Aspiration – aspirate pus (send for MC&S)

Management
- Prophylactic antibiotics (give early, as usually no effect once abscess is formed)
- Refer to surgeons:
  - Incision, drainage and packing
  - Interventional radiology if organ related

Animal bites
Definition
A wound resulting from the teeth of an animal, typically resulting in superficial abrasions, lacerations and puncture wounds. All carry a high risk of bacterial infection.

Epidemiology
Dog and cat bites are commonly treated within urgent and emergency care.

History
- What animal, how and when bite occurred
- First aid given
- Tetanus statues
- Risk factors for infection (i.e. diabetes, immunocompromised)

Examination
- Signs of infection (i.e. redness, heat, swelling, pain, cellulitis, lymphadenopathy, purulent discharge).
- Exclude injury to bone, joints and other deep structures.
- Exclude presence of remaining teeth in wound.

Investigations
- Wound swab for MC&S if signs of infection
- Bloods if septic – U&E, FBC, CRP and blood cultures

Animal bites (continued)
Management
- Thoroughly irrigate wound.
- Consider iodine soaks.
- X-ray if fracture or joint involvement.
- Antibiotic prophylaxis is recommended for:
  - All cat bites
  - Wounds that have been primarily closed
  - Puncture wounds
  - Bites involving face, hands, feet, joints, ligaments and tendons
  - High risk of wound infection (i.e. diabetic, immunocompromised, asplenic or cirrhotic patients and those with prosthetic valves or joints)
- Antibiotics are not usually required if the wound is over 48 hours old and no signs of localised or systemic infection are present.
- Tetanus prophylaxis if required.
- Assess rabies risk (low in the United Kingdom, unless bat bite) and contact HPA (Tel: 020 8327 6017).

Refer to plastic surgery team:

i. Penetrating wounds involving nerves, bones, muscles, tendons, joints and arteries
ii. Presence or possibility of presence of foreign body such as teeth
iii. Facial wounds unless wounds are mild
iv. Bites requiring reconstructive surgery
v. Wounds requiring debridement
vi. People with signs of sepsis or signs of severe cellulitis
vii. Children with scalp wounds (small puncture wound may indicate anchoring of teeth to cranium during shaking – important to identify underlying cranial injury)
viii. Bites to poorly vascularised areas (i.e. nose/ear cartilage)
ix. Wounds requiring closure

Burn to skin
Definition
Injury to the skin caused by heat, flame, radiation (i.e. sunburn), chemicals or electricity.

Epidemiology
More than 12 000 admissions within the UK annually. Commonest types of burns are often caused by flames, hot appliances, scalds and sunburn.

History
How was the burn sustained?
- Cause/type.
- Note time, length of contact and possible temperature.
- Ask about explosions, blasts, burning material and possible loss of consciousness.
- Possible inhalation injury.
- First aid given.
- Ask about tetanus status.

Examination
Airway
- Consider inhalation injury.
- Airway compromise (stridor, hoarse voice).
- Soot in nose and singed nose hair.
- Shortness of breath.

Burn to skin (continued)

Site
- Appearance of burn.
- Capillary refill time (CRT) – a superficial burn CRT will be rapid. CRT will be prolonged in deeper wound.

Pain and sensation
- Severely painful burns are usually less serious as nerve endings are intact. Deeper burns can damage or destroy nerve endings resulting in mild pain/reduced sensation.

Size of burn
- Rule of nines – divides percentage of body surface into multiples of nine:
  - Head 9%, arm 9%, trunk (front) 18%, trunk (back) 18%, legs 18% and perineum 1%

Depth of burn
- Superficial (injury to epidermal layer):
  - Red/glistening, painful, possible blisters and CRT rapid
- Superficial (partial thickness injury to dermal layer):
  - Pink, painful, probably blisters present containing serous fluid. Blisters may burst and skin will be pink/tender and CRT slightly prolonged.
- Deep partial thickness (injury to base of dermal layer, possibly irregular depth):
  - Pale, dry, hair follicles on base of dermal layer may be seen, pain/sensation reduced or absent, CRT very prolonged or absent.
- Full thickness (injury through dermal layer to subcutaneous tissue, muscle or bone):
  - Pale, white, leathery, dry, no blistering, sensation absent and CRT absent

Investigations

Swab for MC&S if signs of infection.
Bloods (if severe):

- U&E, FBC and coagulation
- ABG (note oxygenation and carboxyhaemoglobin)
- X-Match

Management

Severe burns
- ABCDE management.
- Oxygen.
- Early intubation (inhalation injury).
- IV access.
- Fluid resuscitation (consider Muir and Barclay formula if burn >15% or 10% in children).
- Analgesia.
- Anti-emetic.
- Discuss with major trauma centre and regional burns unit.
- Burn should be covered with a sterile dressing.
- Consider antibiotics if signs of infection.
- Tetanus prophylaxis.

Minor burns
- Cool burn (wet compress or under cool running water for 10 minutes).
- Analgesia.
- Clean and dress wounds as appropriate (burn wounds prone to infection).
- Leave blisters intact unless large and located in an awkward position. Aspirate with aseptic technique.

Burn to skin (continued)
- Consider suitable burns dressing (see local policy).
- Review of burn in 24–48 hours.
- If signs of infection present consider antibiotics.
- Tetanus prophylaxis.

Discuss with specialist if:
- Injuries to hands, face, over joints or perineum
- Circumferential
- Signs of inhalation injury
- Superficial burns >1% size
- Suspicious (i.e. non-accidental injury)
- Deep partial thickness or full thickness

Cellulitis
Definition
A bacterial infection of the skin specifically affecting the dermis and subcutaneous fat.

Epidemiology
A common infection caused by streptococcal or staphylococcal organisms which lead to infection via a portal of entry (i.e. a break in the skin). Bites, burns, traumatic wounds and leg ulcers are the main risk factors. Other risk factors include lymphoedema, leg oedema, obesity, venous insufficiency and disruption of lymphatic drainage.

History
- Fever
- Malaise
- Pain, redness, swelling, hot and tender skin
- Often unilateral
- Exposure to fresh or sea water

Examination
- Can be systemically well but in severe infection/sepsis – tachycardia, pyrexia, hypotension, tachypnoea and possible confusion
- Lymphadenopathy
- Diffuse redness or well-demarcated edge
- Break in skin (i.e. laceration or lesion – skin ulcer)
- Blisters/bullae

Investigations
- Swab areas of broken skin.
- Consider FBC and CRP in severe cases.

Management
- Oral antibiotics:
  - If exposed to fresh or sea water a discussion with microbiology may be required.
- Mark area of redness with marker pen if possible to observe further tracking and spread of infection – advise patient that some degree of further tracking is very common.
- Review in 48 hours.
- Analgesia (paracetamol/ibuprofen).
- Elevation of affected area (to promote gravity drainage of the oedema/inflammatory substances and speeds improvement).

Cellulitis (continued)
Consider hospital admission if:

- Unwell with symptoms
- Signs of worsening sepsis
- Under 1 years of age
- Elderly/frail
- Facial cellulitis (unless mild)
- Periorbital cellulitis (refer ophthalmology)
- Immunocompromised
- Severe lymphoedema
- Sinister signs (i.e. possible necrotising fasciitis)

Dermatophyte infection of the skin: Body and groin
Definition
Fungal infection of the skin – often superficial and mild but can be persistent and difficult to eradicate

Also described as tine or ringworm

Commonly seen include:

i. Tine Corpora's – fungal infection of the body
ii. Tine Curries – fungal infection of the groin
iii. Tine Pedi's – fungal infection of the foot

Epidemiology
Common problem see worldwide. Normally associated with direct contact with infected person or animal or indirect contact with items contaminated with the fungus (i.e. clothing)

History
- Commonly itchy red/pink patches
- Direct/indirect contact with infected individual

Examination
- Typically presents as one or more red or pink, flat or slightly raised patches of skin
- Enlarge to become ring-shaped lesions
- Red scaly borders
- Clear central areas

Investigations
MC&S swabs if:

- Infection has not responded to standard topical antifungal treatment.
- Oral antifungals are being considered.
- Diagnosis is unclear.

Note: Samples are not required for mild infections of the skin, feet and groin.

Management
- Topical antifungal treatment for mild non-extensive infection
- Advise person to:
  - Wash affected area daily
  - Wash clothes and bed linen frequently
  - Wear loose fitting clothes
  - Not to share towels and wash towels frequently

Dermatophyte infection of the skin: Body and groin (continued)

In severe or extensive infection:

- Consider oral antifungal treatment.
- Consider referral to dermatologist.
- Seek specialist advice for scalp fungal infections.

Refer immunocompromised people to dermatologist.

Human bite
Definition
A wound resulting from the teeth of a human typically resulting in superficial abrasions, lacerations and puncture wounds. There are two types:

1. Occlusal wound (inflicted by biting)
2. Clenched fist wound (sustained when a clenched fist receives wounds from teeth following punch)

Epidemiology
Actual incidence is not certain but most human bites occur during fighting or through accidental injury associated with sports, contact sports and also during sexual activity.

History
- How and when bite occurred
- First aid given
- Tetanus statues
- Risk factors for infection (i.e. diabetes, immunocompromised)

Examination
- Signs of infection (i.e. redness, heat, swelling, pain, cellulitis, lymphadenopathy, purulent discharge).
- Exclude injury to bone, joints and other deep structures.
- Exclude presence of remaining teeth in wound.

Investigations
- Wound swab for MC&S.
- Seek immediate advice from consultant in microbiology or infectious diseases if person is considered to be at risk from HIV, Hep B or C. Consider all people to be at risk unless statue of the biter is known.
- Consider bloods (FBC, U&E, CRP).

Management
- Thoroughly irrigate wound.
- Consider iodine soaks.
- X-ray if fracture or joint involvement.
- Antibiotic prophylaxis is recommended for:
- Tetanus prophylaxis if required (rare with human bites).

Refer to plastic surgery:

- Penetrating wounds involving nerves, bones, muscles, tendons, joints and arteries
- Presence or possibility of presence of foreign body such as teeth
- Facial wounds unless wounds are mild
- Bites requiring reconstructive surgery
- Wounds requiring debridement
- People with signs of sepsis
- Wounds with signs of severe cellulitis

Human bite (continued)
- Bites to poorly vascularised areas (i.e. nose/ear cartilage)
- Wounds requiring closure

Impetigo
Definition
Highly contagious bacterial superficial skin infection.
  There are two types:

1. Non-bullous – often caused by staphylococcal or streptococcal organisms
2. Bullous (less common) – often caused by staphylococcal organisms

Epidemiology
Can affect any age but predominantly affects children. Those who play close contact sports (i.e. rugby) are also susceptible.

History
- Non-healing crusty lesion(s).
- Lesions can be itchy (non-bullous).
- Painful lesions (bullous).
- Regional lymphadenopathy.
- Weakness, fever and diarrhoea (bullous).
- Outbreak in schools, nurseries, etc.

Examination
Non-bullous – lesions begin as vesicles/pustules, commonly around mouth/nose. Rapidly develops into gold crusty plaques. Satellite lesions can be present. Often asymptomatic.
Bullous – flaccid fluid-filled vesicles/blisters. Often burst and form flat brown to golden crusts. Commonly affects neonates around axillae, skin folds and nappy areas. Systemic symptoms (i.e. fever) can be present.

Investigations
- Skin swabs are not routinely required.
- Obtain a skin swab if the infection is:
  - Extensive
  - Recurrent
  - Suspected of MRSA
  - During community outbreak
  - Not resolved after 7 days' treatment

Management
- Topical antibiotics for very localised lesions.
- Oral antibiotics for extensive, severe or bullous impetigo.
- Educate patient regarding good hand washing technique and avoid itching to improve healing and helps to avoid further transmission.

Necrotising fasciitis
Definition
Commonly a group A streptococcal or polymicrobial with streptococci, staphylococci, bacteroides and coliforms, which is rapidly progressive and destructive. Infection of the deep subcutaneous tissue and fascia.

Epidemiology
A rare condition that can affect any age. Approximately half of the people who develop necrotising fasciitis will die from it.

Necrotising fasciitis (continued)
History
- Fever
- Malaise
- Pain, often severe and out of proportion
- Diarrhoea and vomiting
- Possible recent surgery, trauma or ulceration

Examination
- Often mistaken for cellulitis (redness, swelling, tender skin)
- Tachycardia, pyrexia, hypotension and tachypnoea
- Confusion/delirium
- Break in skin
- Intense pain that appears out of proportion to external signs of infection to skin
- Pyrexia
- Oedema
- Reduced skin sensation
- Bruise-type blotches
- Bullae
- Skin necrosis
- Firm feeling to subcutaneous tissue

Investigations
- Bloods (FBC, U&E, CRP, cultures and ABG)
- Wound swab for MC&S
- Radiology

Management
- Urgent referral to plastic surgery.
- Admit to hospital and discuss with ICU.
- Oxygen if required.
- IV access.
- Fluid resuscitation.
- Analgesia.
- Antibiotics (broad spectrum).

Scabies
Definition
Intensely itchy skin infestation caused by the human parasite *Sarcoptes scabiei*. There are two types: classical scabies and crusted scabies (hyperinfestation due to immunocompromised; appears hyperkeratotic resembling psoriasis).

Epidemiology
Estimated 300 million cases worldwide each year. **More common in urban areas, in the north of the United Kingdom, during winter and in women and children**. Scabies can spread easily between close contact of people.

History
- Generalised itchy rash.
- Occasionally no itch present. Young children may present with no history of itch but do not appear to be themselves.
- Itching worse at night.
- Contact with another person with scabies or similar symptoms.

Scabies (continued)
Examination
- Silvery lines in skin where mites have burrowed.
- Red vesicular or papular lesions often around silvery lines.
- Typical sites include hands, wrists, elbows and nipples (females).

Crusted scabies appears different to classical scabies. Features include:

- Redness and scaling to the face, neck and scalp.
- Silvery lines of burrows may be difficult to see.
- Thickened horny honeycombed layers which contain large numbers of mites.
- Palms and soles may have deep fissuring of the crusts.
- Nail hyperkeratosis is common.
- Commonly secondary bacterial infection.
- Possible generalised lymphadenopathy.
- Possibly localised to one particular area.

Investigations
- Confirming presence of mite is not required for diagnosis of classical scabies.
- Skin scraping will be required for crusted scabies.

Management
- Topical insecticides.
- Consider treatment for itch (i.e. antihistamine).
- Treat all household/sexual contacts within 24 hours even in absence of symptoms.
- Machine wash (above 50°C) all towels/bed linen/clothes on day of topical application.
- Consider referral to dermatologist if diagnosis uncertain or if treatment failure after two courses of insecticide.

Note
- Seek specialist advice from dermatologist if anyone presents with crusted scabies.
- Scabies is rare in children under 2 months of age. Seek specialist advice from paediatrician/dermatologist if treatment is required in this age group.
- Consider referral to genito-urinary clinic if there is a history of risk sexual behaviour.

Varicella infection
Definition
A herpesvirus – varicella zoster (chickenpox) and herpes zoster (shingles)

Epidemiology
Varicella zoster – predominantly seen in children <10 years of age. Peak incidence often occurs between March and May.

Herpes zoster – occurs when varicella zoster virus is reactivated from latency in the central nervous system. Exact prevalence unknown but commonly seen in primary care.

History
Varicella zoster – fever, malaise, nausea, headache, itchy red spotty rash and possible contact with infected individual

Herpes zoster – burning, tingling, pruritus and numbness over area of affected skin several days before rash occurs; area of painful rash; possible contact with infected individual

Examination
Varicella zoster – fever, rash, widespread vesicular lesions and often in varying stages of development

Herpes zoster – vesicular lesions in a dermatomal distribution

Varicella infection (continued)
Investigations
Diagnosis is made on clinical grounds.

Management
Varicella zoster
- Analgesia.
- Consider topical lotions/antihistamine for itch relief.
- Encourage adequate fluid intake.
- Consider antiviral medication if >14, present within 24 hours of rash, in severe pain, dense oral rash, secondary household case, prescribed steroids or is a smoker.
- Refer to specialist if person is immunocompromised, signs of ophthalmic involvement, pneumonia or encephalitis.
- Avoid contact with immunocompromised people, neonates and pregnant women.
- If pregnant or breastfeeding seek specialist advice.

Herpes zoster
- Analgesia.
- Start antiviral medication within 72 hours of onset of rash for anyone >50 years, presence of non-truncal involvement or those in moderate or severe pain.
- Consider starting antiviral medication if presenting with rash >7 days and are at higher risk of complications/severe shingles.
- Always treat if active ophthalmic involvement, Ramsay Hunt syndrome or eczema.
- Seek specialist advice if person has had two episodes or if any signs of ophthalmic involvement or is immunocompromised.
- Avoid contact with immunocompromised people, neonates and pregnant women.
- If pregnant or breastfeeding seek specialist advice.

The electrocardiogram

Rapid Emergency and Unscheduled Care, First Edition. Oliver Phipps and Jason Lugg.
© 2016 John Wiley & Sons, Ltd. Published 2016 by John Wiley & Sons, Ltd.

Electrocardiograph (ECG)

ECG component	Normal value (s)
P wave	0.10
QRS complex	<0.12
T wave	0.15–0.25
PR interval	0.12–0.20
ST segment	0.2

Atrial fibrillation
Definition
Disorganised atrial activity, with an inconsistent ventricular response.

Characteristics
Rate: ventricular rate 60–160 per minute
Rhythm: irregular
P waves: none seen
PR interval: can't interpret
QRS complex: normal

Significance
AF can be caused by underlying disease including heart disease, mitral valve disease, alcohol, drugs, dehydration, medicine (digoxin), hypoxia, infection, thyrotoxicosis and cardiac surgery. A rapid rate may lead to hypotension and hypoperfusion leading to chest pain, caused by reduced cardiac output. Patients in AF often require anticoagulation.

Atrial flutter
Definition
Atrial depolarisation is driven by electrical activity which is independent to SA node activity. This gives a 'sawtooth' appearance on the ECG known as F waves. The ventricles are unable to respond to such a fast rate so the AV node blocks them. This results in more F waves than QRS complexes.

Characteristics
Rate: atrial rate 220–350 per minute (ventricular rate depends on AV block)
Rhythm: atrial regular (ventricular can be irregular or regular)
P waves: none seen
PR interval: can't interpret
QRS complex: normal

Significance
Flutter can be caused by underlying heart disease, congestive cardiac failure and increased sympathetic tone. A rapid rate may lead to hypotension and hypoperfusion leading to chest pain, which is caused by reduced cardiac output.

Asystole
Definition
No electrical activity

Characteristics
Rate: none
Rhythm: none
P waves: none
PR interval: can't interpret
QRS complex: none

Significance
Advanced life support (CPR) is required. This will be fatal if left untreated.

First-degree heart block
Definition
Originating in the SA node, the impulse is slowed through the AV node which results in longer PR interval.

Characteristics
Rate: 60–100 per minute
Rhythm: regular
P waves: normal
PR interval: >200 ms
QRS complex: normal

Significance
Causes include node damage, increased vagal tone, hypoxia and drug toxicity. This usually has no significance.

Normal sinus rhythm
Definition
A normal rhythm, where each P wave is followed by a QRS complex

Characteristics
Rate: 60–100 per minute
Rhythm: regular
P waves: preceding each QRS
QRS complex: normal

Significance
This is a normal rhythm.

Pulseless electrical activity (PEA)
Definition
QRS complexes can be seen, but no palpable pulse is felt.

Characteristics
Rate: variable
Rhythm: regular and irregular
P waves: yes and no
PR interval: can be seen
QRS complex: normal or wide

Pulseless electrical activity (PEA) (continued)
Significance
Advanced life support (CPR) is required. This will be fatal if left untreated. Focus on treating the 4H's and 4T's (hypoxia, hypovolaemia, hypothermia, hypo-/hyperkalaemia, tension pneumothorax, cardiac tamponade, toxins and thrombus).

Second-degree heart block: Mobitz type 1 (Wenckebach)
Definition
Conduction is delayed at AV node for a longer time each cycle, appearing as an increasing PR interval, until a beat/complex is dropped.

Characteristics
Rate: normal or slow
Rhythm: atrial regular, ventricular irregular
P waves: normal
PR interval: progressively increasing until a beat is dropped
QRS complex: normal

Significance
Causes include node damage, increased vagal tone, hypoxia and drug toxicity. May be little or no clinical significance unless rate is slow. Hypotension, hypoperfusion and hypoxia can occur.

Second-degree heart block: Mobitz type 2
Definition
Like type 1, but the AV node conducts most impulses, but blocks every second, third, fourth, etc. Described as 2:1, 3:1, 4:1 block.

Characteristics
Rate: normal or slow
Rhythm: atrial regular, ventricular regularly irregular
P waves: normal
PR interval: some P waves not followed by QRS complexes
QRS complex: normal or widened

Significance
Causes include node damage, increased vagal tone, hypoxia and drug toxicity. Hypotension, hypoperfusion and hypoxia can occur.
  Can progress to complete heart block.

Sinus bradycardia
Definition
Slower rate than normal.

Characteristics
Rate: <60 per minute
Rhythm: regular
P waves: preceding each QRS
QRS complex: normal

Significance
This may be normal in young fit adults. However it could be as a result of hypoxia, brain injury or overdose. This slow rate may cause hypotension, confusion and poor tissue perfusion.

Sinus tachycardia
Definition
A faster rate than normal, with a QRS complex following each P wave.

Characteristics
Rate: >100 per minute
Rhythm: regular
P waves: preceding each QRS, but may be hidden in T wave if very fast
QRS complex: normal

Significance
This would be a normal response to vigorous exercise but could be caused by anxiety, pain, fever, shock and hypoxia.

Supraventricular tachycardia (SVT)
Definition
The pacemaker is above the ventricles in the atria, SA or VA nodes.

Characteristics
Rate: ventricular rate 150–220 per minute
Rhythm: regular
P waves: absent
PR interval: can't interpret
QRS complex: normal

Significance
SVT is caused by idiopathic, damage to nodes, drug overdose, sympathetic stimuli, caffeine, etc. Can cause hypotension, hypoperfusion and hypoxia. Chest pain is likely caused by myocardial ischemia.

Third-degree heart block: Complete heart block
Definition
A disassociation between the atria and ventricles, caused by an AV node failure.

Characteristics
Rate: atrial normal, ventricular 20–40 per minute
Rhythm: atrial regular, ventricular regular
P waves: normal, can be hidden in QRS
PR interval: disassociation between P waves and QRS complexes
QRS complex: normal or broad

Significance
Poor cardiac output caused by a slow ventricular rate. Hypotension and hypoperfusion can occur leading to ventricular fibrillation and ventricular standstill.

Torsade de pointes
Definition
A form of ventricular tachycardia, where antiarrhythmic drugs can cause an adverse effect.

Characteristics
Irregular and bizarre, with the waveform appearing to change amplitude.

Significance
Hypoperfusion and hypotension can occur. Often cardioversion is required and IV magnesium is recommended.

Ventricular fibrillation
Definition
Uncoordinated and disassociated, with large numbers of myocardial cells depolarising and repolarising asynchronously.

Characteristics
Rate: variable
Rhythm: irregular
P waves: none
PR interval: not seen
QRS complex: none

Significance
Advanced life support (CPR and defibrillation) is required. This will be fatal if left untreated.

Ventricular standstill
Definition
No ventricular activity

Characteristics
Rate: no ventricular rate
Rhythm: absent
P waves: normal
PR interval: not seen
QRS complex: none

Significance
Advanced life support (CPR) is required. This will be fatal if left untreated.

Ventricular tachycardia (VT)
Definition
Impulse starts in the ventricles and rate is around 200–300 per minute. If no pulse present this is 'pulseless VT' and ALS/CPR should begin.

Characteristics
Rate: 200–300 per minute
Rhythm: irregular/regular
P waves: none
PR interval: not seen
QRS complex: wide and bizarre

Significance
If no pulse, advanced life support (CPR and defibrillation) is required and will be fatal if left untreated. If pulse present/conscious hypotension and hypoperfusion are likely.

Index

Rapid Emergency and Unscheduled Care, First Edition. Oliver Phipps and Jason Lugg.
© 2016 John Wiley & Sons, Ltd. Published 2016 by John Wiley & Sons, Ltd.